Health Essentials

Chinese Medicine

Tom Williams Ph.D. is a practising acupuncturist and Member
of the Register of Traditional Chinese Medicine. As well
as being a Senior Educational Psychologist in Ayrshire,
Scotland, he is Regional Tutor for the Northern College
of Acupuncture and a tutor counsellor in social sciences with
the Open University.

The Health Essentials Series

There is a growing number of people who find themselves attracted to holistic or alternative therapies and natural approaches to maintaining optimum health and vitality. The *Health Essentials* series is designed to help the newcomer by presenting high quality introductions to all the main complementary health subjects. Each book presents all the essential information on each therapy, explaining what it is, how it works and what it can do for the reader. Advice is also given, where possible, on how to begin using the therapy at home, together with comprehensive lists of courses and classes available worldwide.

The *Health Essentials* titles are all written by practising experts in their fields. Exceptionally clear and concise, each text is supported by attractive illustrations.

Series Medical Consultant
Dr John Cosh MD, FRCP

In the same series

Acupuncture by Peter Mole
Alexander Technique by Richard Brennan
Aromatherapy by Christine Wildwood
Ayurveda by Scott Gerson
Chi Kung by James MacRitchie
Colour Therapy by Pauline Wills
Flower Remedies by Christine Wildwood
Herbal Medicine by Vicki Pitman
Kinesiology by Ann Holdway
Massage by Stewart Mitchell
Reflexology by Inge Dougans with Suzanne Ellis
Shiatsu by Elaine Liechti
Skin and Body Care by Sidra Shaukat
Spiritual Healing by Jack Angelo
Vitamin Guide by Hasnain Walji

Health Essentials

CHINESE MEDICINE

Acupuncture, Herbal Remedies, Nutrition, Qigong and Meditation for Total Health

TOM WILLIAMS

E L E M E N T

Shaftesbury, Dorset ● Rockport, Massachusetts
Brisbane, Queensland

© Tom Williams 1995

First published in Great Britain in 1995 by
Element Books Limited
Shaftesbury, Dorset SP7 8BP

Published in the USA in 1995 by
Element Books, Inc.
PO Box 830, Rockport, MA 01966

Published in Australia in 1995 by
Element Books Limited
for Jacaranda Wiley Limited
33 Park Road, Milton, Brisbane, 4064

Reprinted November 1995

Cover design by Max Fairbrother
Page design by Roger Lightfoot
Typeset by The Electronic Book Factory Ltd, Fife
Printed and bound in Great Britain by
Biddles Ltd, Guildford and King's Lynn

British Library Cataloguing in Publication

Library of Congress Cataloguing in Publication
Williams, Tom, 1948–
Chinese Medicine/Tom Williams.
P. cm. – (Health Essentials series)
Includes bibliographical references and index.
ISBN 1–85230–589–4
1. Medicine. Chinese. I. Title. II. Series.
R601. W55 1995
610Y. 951– dc20 94-47044

Note from the Publisher

Any information given in any book in the *Health Essentials*
series is not intended to be taken as a replacement for medical
advice. Any person with a condition requiring medical attention should consult a qualified medical practitioner or suitable
therapist.

Contents

Foreword

CHINESE MEDICINE, BOTH in its philosophical content as well as in its practical application to the healing of disease, has a great deal to offer the Western mind. First and foremost, Chinese medicine operates from the perception that illness is created as a consequence of a disturbance occurring within a person's emotional and mental bodies. Western medicine still neglects this truth. Secondly, Chinese medicine philosophically maintains that healing is a process that must engage the entire body – that is, regardless of where in the physical body an illness has developed, the understanding is that the entire body is ill. Western medicine still maintains that a disease is an isolated entity in a body – thus, statements such as 'the cancer is contained in this organ' are commonly heard in our hospitals. The Chinese perception is the accurate one – when illness develops, regardless of what it is and where it locates itself – the fact is that the entire body is ill.

The Western medical world, and the population on this side of the globe, has much to learn from Chinese medicine. Chinese medicine brims over with wisdom, logic and a deeply thorough understanding of the full content of what it means to be a thinking, feeling human being. The language used to describe both the human being and the illness, while often symbolic, is also incredibly more on target. For example, according to Chinese medicine, we are made up of earth, wind, fire, water and metal. Translated into practical terms, people who have too much water are often more emotional and prone to depression and other illnesses that are the consequence of the mismanagement of one's water content. Too much fire in a person causes a hot temper and the illnesses produced by too much fire feel like fire – migraine headaches, neurological disorders and rheumatoid arthritis – all burning diseases. Fire disorders are treated with water remedies because fire needs to be cooled. Too much air and not enough earth results in a person who has an abundance of ideas and an insufficient amount of patience to bring these ideas to fruition. Impatience and nervousness manifest in a person with too much air in his or her nature. The treatment: earth remedies, assisting in grounding the person.

This book comes at the right time. The Western world is more than ready to add to its own technical medical knowledge the wisdom that comes from working with the spirit of the human being in order to heal the body.

Caroline M. Myss, MA
International teacher, lecturer and
author of *Creation of Health –
Merging Traditional Medicine with
Intuitive Diagnosis* with C. Norman
Shealy, MD, Ph.D.

Acknowledgements

THERE ARE MANY people who deserve to be mentioned and without whom I would never have had the confidence to attempt this book. Firstly, I must mention my teachers of Chinese medicine who have become more than passers-on of information; they are now more fellow travellers on the same journey. To Hugh McPherson, Richard Blackwell, Nick Haines, Charlie Buck and Han Liping, thank you for bringing the gift of Chinese medicine to me. Secondly, there are many friends who have helped me believe in myself and with whom I have been able to share some of the insights of Chinese medicine. Gabrielle McGuire has demonstrated the reality of Qi energy; Gillian Kamming has been my closest 'ear' about so many things; George Docherty has made me laugh till I dropped. To all of them and many others beyond mention – thanks. To all my patients and students – past, present and future – a sincere thanks. I have learned something unique from all of you.

I have to pay especial thanks to Caroline Myss, not only a wonderful teacher but also one of the most inspirational and visionary figures in the field of energy medicine in the world today. Caroline's contribution will probably never be fully grasped until long after we are all gone, but her friendship, knowledge, encouragement and professionalism have been a constant source of inspiration to me.

Finally, of course, a heartfelt sense of love and thanks to my family – Mary, Emma, Jennifer and Neil – your patience and understanding are without limits.

I dedicate this book to my wife Mary: a better example of true healing energy, both personally and professionally, it would be hard to find.

An Introduction to Chinese Medicine

CHINESE MEDICINE IS a system of diagnosis and health-care approaches that have evolved over the last 3000 years. The Chinese approach to understanding the human body is unique and is based on the holistic understanding of the universe as outlined in the spiritual insights of Daoism. This understanding has produced a highly sophisticated set of practices designed to cure illness and to maintain health and well-being. These practices, including acupuncture, herbal remedies, diet, meditation and both static and moving exercises, appear very different in approach yet they all share the same underlying sets of assumptions and insights into the nature of the human body and its place in the universe.

The last twenty years or so have seen a dramatic increase in the popularity of a whole range of therapies that have their origins well outside the accepted boundaries of Western scientific thought. The derivatives of Chinese medicine – particularly acupuncture, herbal remedies and Qigong exercises – have been among the most notable and they now enjoy a growing respect not only from patients who have experienced their benefits at first hand but also from an initially sceptical Western medical fraternity.

However, regardless of the therapeutic benefits, it is likely that patients will, at some point in the process, ask themselves the question 'How is this working?' On face value, it is only common sense to wonder why the insertion of fine needles into a variety of points on the body – more often than not bearing no obvious relationship to the presenting problem – can have such a dramatic effect. Any patient wrestling with the problem of trying to consume a herbal mixture that would do justice to the witches in Macbeth must, at times, question what is going on. Many hundreds of practitioners who experience for themselves the

1

benefits of Chinese 'Soft Exercises' – Taiqi, Qigong and so on – find themselves wondering how these therapies differ from traditional aerobic Western-oriented exercise. Yet, in all cases, the proof is there in terms of symptomatic relief, improved health and well-being and, often, a more balanced view of life in general.

This book will seek to try and provide answers to some of these questions.

- What is this body of knowledge that has remained hidden in China for almost 3000 years and that is now having such an impact throughout the Western world?
- How does the Chinese system differ from the systems we are so used to in the West?
- How would a practitioner use this body of knowledge in a systematic manner in order to understand a patient's problem and to plan an appropriate course of treatment?
- What lessons does this Chinese system have for the way in which medicine is practised in the West as we move towards the end of the millennium?

A HISTORICAL OVERVIEW

It is worth spending a short time looking at the growth and development of Chinese medicine over the centuries in order to provide a contextual backdrop for the discussions in this book.

There is evidence dating back to the Shang Dynasty (c.1000BC) that there was already a relatively sophisticated approach to medical problems. Archaeological diggings have unearthed early types of acupuncture needle and the discussion of medical conditions has been found inscribed on bones dating back to this time.

In keeping with the Chinese emphasis on the balancing and governing forces of nature, it seems likely that such practices developed through the observation of the natural world. Many of the graceful postures in Taiqi and Qigong relate to the observation of animal behaviour. For example, the various movements of wild geese form the basis for Dayan Qigong, which relates the movements in human terms to the acupuncture points and the energy body. There is clear evidence of a Shamanic culture existing in early Asian civilization and many Shamanic practices are believed to be at the foundation of Chinese medicine. By the sixth century BC, the link between the Shaman and the medical practitioner was clear. Confucius is quoted as

2

saying that 'a man without persistence will never make a good shaman or a good physician'.[1]

Both acupuncture and massage practices developed in an empirical manner through the observation of the effects they produced on certain parts of the body and on specific internal ailments. Early acupuncture was carried out using sharpened bone fragments prior to the development of other tools.

By the first century AD the first and most important classic text of Chinese medicine had been completed. This work, probably compiled over several centuries by various authors, takes the form of a dialogue between the legendary Yellow Emperor and his minister Qi Bo, on the topic of medicine. This book – known as the *Inner Classic* – discusses the theory and philosophy of Chinese medicine in one section (*Basic Questions*) and goes on to expand on the therapeutic benefits of acupuncture, herbs, diet and exercise in the second section (*Miraculous Pivot*).[2] Over the following centuries, these basic classics were expanded and specific works emerged on acupuncture, for example *The Systematic Classic of Acupuncture & Moxabustion*[3] – and on herbal remedies, for example *The Divine Husbandman's Classic of the Materia Medica*.[4] Right into the twentieth century much of the practice of Chinese medicine reflected the traditions that had developed over the preceding 3000 years.

However, Western culture was also making an impact in China, driven by the colonial expansionism of the previous few centuries. The initial response, however, was for the more traditional ancient theories based on Yin and Yang and Five Elements to withdraw under the weight of Western scientific determinism. By the time the communists took power in China in 1949, there was a real dilemma regarding how best to deal with the apparent dichotomy between Western-based medical practices and those of the traditional practitioners.

By 1954, the government officially recognized traditional practitioners as representing a 'medical legacy of the motherland' and thus began what became an ostensibly dual-track process of developing Western medical practices in parallel with Chinese medical practices.

A process was set in motion that brought together the diverse practices of the centuries into a recognizable modern curriculum of Chinese medicine. While much of this process became muddied with the ideology and dogma of the cultural revolution, nonetheless, a coherent body of knowledge has appeared under the generic descriptor of traditional Chinese medicine. In order to avoid debates on what constitutes traditional and what doesn't, we will work with the general understanding that what is being described is simply – Chinese medicine.

As these texts from the major teaching centres in China have been translated and made available in the West, there has been a parallel process that has sought to make the ideas, principles and practices more accessible to the Western reader. Many Western practitioners have written invaluable teaching texts aimed at the Western student of Chinese medicine, while some other writers have sought to bring the ideas to a more general audience. This short book hopefully continues this trend, by seeking to make the ideas, principles and practices accessible to the interested lay reader in a manner that will allow a greater understanding and appreciation of the rich knowledge base that guides the practitioner of Chinese medicine in today's eclectic and cosmopolitan society.

CHINESE MEDICINE IN THE FUTURE

Clearly it is necessary to step back into the past to understand where Chinese medicine has come from and to understand how it links with ancient philosophical thinking, but this book is about helping people to understand Chinese medicine in today's Western industrialized society and to suggest the place that it can rightly occupy in the developing medicine and health care of the twenty-first century.

Patients will more and more come to expect that when they put themselves in the hands of professional health-care workers, whether it is a Western-trained doctor or a practitioner of Chinese medicine, they will be offered an explanation about what is being done and why. This is as it should be and this book aims to equip patients with enough basic understanding so that they will not feel confused when talking with their Chinese medical practitioner.

This is a fascinating and enthralling journey. You will be asked to view your world from a very different perspective, but once you get used to the new landscape the view can be breathtaking and the rewards, in terms of your health, second to none.

Read on and enjoy!

1

The Basic Principles Behind Chinese Medicine

W HEN WE THINK of medical practices in the West we make the valid assumption that the skills of the doctor are founded on well-researched science regarding how the body works and what mechanisms can go wrong in the course of illness. Thus, the practice of medicine as the patient experiences it is based on a firm foundation of scientific principle.

However, it is equally important to understand that the subtlety and complexities of Chinese medicine are based on firm philosophies and principles, which while differing dramatically from those in the West, are nonetheless rigorous and valid for that. In beginning to understand what Chinese medicine is all about it is important firstly to explore this different frame of reference. Without this, the system the Chinese use to understand the body's harmonies and disharmonies will seem like ad hoc mumbo jumbo designed to confuse rather than to enlighten.

YIN AND YANG

The concept behind Yin and Yang is beyond question the most important and the most fundamental with regard to understanding Chinese medicine. The ideas behind Yin and Yang developed from observing all aspects of the physical world. It was observed that nature appears to group into pairs of mutually dependent opposites. Thus, for example, the concept of 'night' has no meaning without the concept of 'day', the concept of 'up' has no meaning without a concept of 'down' and so on.

5

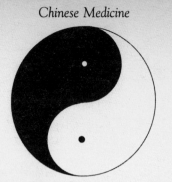

Figure 1. The Yin/Yang symbol – the Taiji

The implications of this apparently straightforward observation leads us in a direction quite at odds with the Aristotelian logic that underpins Western scientific thought. To take a simple example. In Western thought a circle is a circle and it is not a square. Measurement and properties define it as a circle. However, from the Chinese perspective of Yin and Yang, a circle contains within it the potential of a square and vice versa and thus dichotomies would be avoided.

Yin and Yang are represented by the universally recognized, yet rarely understood symbol (see Figure 1).

In keeping with the Chinese emphasis on process rather than structure – a topic that will be revisited time and again in the course of our discussions – it is important to understand the concept that Yin and Yang are essentially descriptors of the dynamic interactions that underpin all aspects of the universe. Thus, Yin and Yang should not be seen as 'things' in the true Western sense of the term, but as a system of thinking about the world.

The Chinese characters give a sense of this (see Figures 2 and 3). The character for Yin translates literally as the 'dark side of the mountain' and represents such qualities as cold, stillness, passive, dark, within, potential and so on. The character for Yang translates literally as the 'bright side of the mountain' and represents such qualities as warmth, activity, light, outside, expression and so on.

This way of thinking about the world leads to certain underlying

Figure 2. The character for Yin

Figure 3. The character for Yang

principles relating to Yin and Yang. In the following descriptions of each, we will see how these can be shown to relate to the Chinese view of the human body and its functioning.

All Things in the Universe Contain Yin and Yang Aspects

It would be true to say that according to the Chinese view, everything has existence in the physical exactly because everything manifests both Yin and Yang qualities. The relative emphasis of Yin and Yang will vary, but both aspects are always present. For example, in viewing the organs of the body, the Chinese system emphasizes the two qualities. The Liver is generally considered a Yin organ as it is quite solid, but it also has the function of promoting Qi flow (see Chapter 2), so to that extent it has a Yang quality. The stomach on the other hand is hollow and moves food through it, so is thus considered Yang. However, it also has a storing aspect that will represent the Yin function. All these aspects of Yin and Yang are fundamentally interdependent.

Within Yin and Yang, Further Aspects of Yin and Yang Can Be Identified

In theory all Yin and Yang can be infinitely subdivided into aspects that are themselves Yin and Yang. Steam, for example, would be considered a Yang quality of water, whereas ice would be considered a Yin quality. However, both steam and ice can be seen in terms of water molecules that themselves have Yin particles – protons and neutrons – in relation to Yang particles – electrons. No doubt if we delved further into quantum physics we would see further aspects of Yin and Yang appearing. In Chinese medicine, the front of the body is considered Yin in relation to the back, which is Yang, but the upper part of the front – the chest – would be seen as Yang in relation to the lower part of the front – the abdomen.

7

Yin Transforms into Yang and Yang Transforms into Yin

The mutual interdependence of Yin and Yang point to the dynamic interaction between the two. Change is at the root of all things and this change manifests itself as Yang transforming into Yin and vice versa. If the Yin and Yang aspects are prevented from achieving balance through this mutual transformation process then the consequences may be catastrophic as, ultimately, balance will be achieved.

For example, the efficient functioning of a tyre depends on a balance between the pressure in the tyre and the strength of the tyre wall. Balance will always be achieved, but if the pressure is too low, the tyre will not perform its function, whereas if it is too high, then balance will be achieved through a catastrophic interchange of Yin and Yang as the tyre bursts. To take an example from human health, if someone is suffering from a fever then this is seen as a relative excess of Yang in Chinese medicine. The principle of treatment will be to allow the transformation of the excess Yang into Yin in order to re-establish equilibrium and biological homoeostasis. Thus, the fever would break and the temperature would begin to return to normal – Yang transforming into Yin. It is also interesting to note that the early manifestation of a fever is likely to be seen as a relative excess of Yin with chills and cold signs. As the condition develops, then the Yin transforms into Yang and the fever develops.

Chinese medicine views the body in terms of Yin and Yang aspects. The healthy state is characterized by a dynamic balance between the Yin and Yang aspects of the body and, by implication, an unhealthy state is characterized by some imbalance between the Yin and Yang of the body.

Essentially all disharmonies can be reduced to a relative imbalance of Yin and Yang (see Figure 4). Thus:

Figure 4(a) illustrates an actual excess of Yin and will be characterized by extreme cold symptoms. Figure 4(b) illustrates an actual excess of Yang and will be characterized by very full heat symptoms. Figure 4(c) illustrates a relative deficiency of Yin and will be characterized by internal heat and lethargy symptoms. Figure 4(d) illustrates a relative deficiency of Yang and will be characterized by general coldness and lethargy symptoms. Figure 4(e) represents the ideal balance state of health where Yin and Yang are in dynamic equilibrium.

These patterns will be discussed later in greater detail, but at present they serve to illustrate the importance of Yin and Yang in understanding body process.

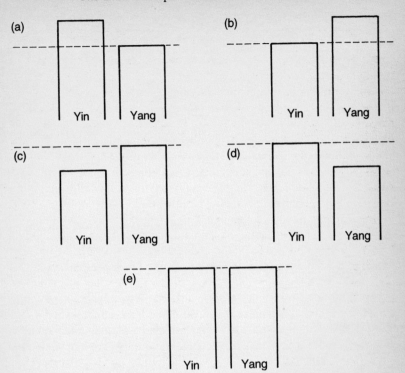

Figure 4. Yin and Yang in harmony or disharmony?

THE FIVE ELEMENTS IN CHINESE MEDICINE

The philosophical origins of all Chinese thinking in general, and Chinese medicine in particular, have grown out of the tenets of Daoism (often written as 'Taoism'). Daoism bases much of its thinking on observing the natural world and the manner in which it operates. In Chinese medicine, this leads to a metaphoric view of the human body based on observation of Yin and Yang interchanges in the natural world. The Chinese observed that everywhere there is dynamic interchange. The seed (Yin) grows into the plant (Yang), which itself dies back into the earth (Yin). This takes place within the changes of the seasons – Winter (Yin) transforms through the Spring into Summer (Yang), which in turn transforms through the Autumn into Winter again. It is no surprise then to find the Chinese medical system drawing extensively on natural metaphors. This is most fully articulated in the system of the 'Five Elements' or 'Five Phases'.

The Five Elements emerged from an observation of the various

9

groups of dynamic processes, functions and characteristics observed in the natural world. They are:

1. **Water:** wet, cool, descending, flowing, yielding and so on.
2. **Fire:** dry, hot, ascending, moving and so on.
3. **Wood:** growing, flexible, rooted, strong and so on.
4. **Metal:** cutting, hard, conducting and so on.
5. **Earth:** productive, fertile, potential for growth and so on.

These characteristics are merely exemplars of how the elements can be seen, but the important feature is that all of them will contain both Yin and Yang aspects, thus reflecting this underlying principle of mutually interactive duality, so central to Chinese thought.

Each Element is seen as having a series of correspondences relating both to the natural world and also the human body. These correspondences can be summarized in the opposite table (see Figure 5).

Chinese medicine uses a system of inter-relationships between the Five Elements in order to understand how the various processes of the body support and control each other. These inter-relationships are defined through the Sheng and the Ke cycles.

The Sheng Cycle – The Cycle of Mutual Production or Promotion

This cycle (Figure 6) represents the manner in which the elements – and by implication the organ systems of the body – support and promote one another. Thus, for example, Fire burns to create Earth, Water nourishes the growth of Wood and so on. When Chinese medicine applies this promotion cycle to the organ system then similar promotional relationships develop. Thus:

● The Heart supports the Spleen.
● The Spleen supports the Lungs.
● The Lungs support the Kidneys.
● The Kidneys support the Liver.
● The Liver supports the Heart.

This promotion cycle is sometimes referred to as the 'Mother and Son' cycle. Thus, for example, the Kidney would be the 'mother' to her 'son', the Liver. A common example of this in Chinese medicine would be when the Kidney Yin energy is deficient, then this often leads to the Liver Yin energy also being deficient. Also, in treatment terms, the 'mother' can be used to treat the 'son'. So, if the Lung energy was deficient then this could be treated by tonifying the Spleen, for example.

	Wood	Fire	Earth	Metal	Water
Season	Spring	Summer	Late Summer	Autumn	Winter
Direction	East	South	Centre	West	North
Climate	Wind	Heat	Dampness	Dryness	Cold
Colour	Blue/green	Red	Yellow	White	Blue/black
Taste	Sour	Bitter	Sweet	Pungent	Salty
Smell	Rancid	Burnt	Fragrant	Rotting	Putrid
Yin organ (Zang)	Liver	Heart	Spleen	Lungs	Kidney
Yang organ (Fu)	Gall bladder	Small intestine	Stomach	Large intestine	Bladder
Orifice	Eyes	Tongue	Mouth	Nose	Ears
Tissue	Tendons	Blood vessels	Muscles	Skin	Bones
Emotion	Anger	Joy	Pensiveness	Grief	Fear
Voice	Shout	Laugh	Sing	Weep	Groan

Figure 5. Five Elements' table of correspondences

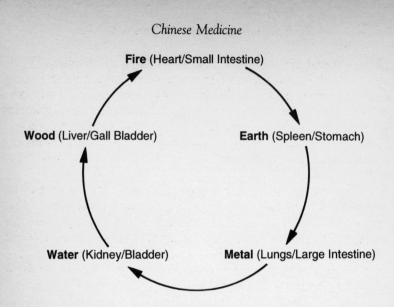

Figure 6. *The Sheng cycle: how the Five Elements can support each other*

The Ke Cycle – The Cycle of Mutual Control

This set of relationships (Figure 7) refers to the observed manner in which the Elements in the natural world control each other as part of the process of dynamic equilibrium. Thus, for example, Fire will

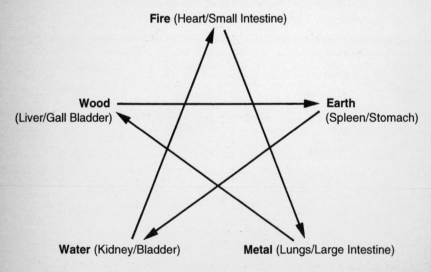

Figure 7. *The Ke cycle: how the Five Elements can control each other*

'control' Metal in the sense that fire will melt metal. Similarly, Water will 'control' Fire in the sense that water can dampen down fire. In terms of Chinese medicine, the notion of control is seen as part of the process of one organ assisting the process of another. For example, the Lung will help to 'control' the Liver energy, thus assisting the smooth function of the Liver. When a disharmony occurs, a weak organ may be unable to exert the control and assistance necessary for another organ.

Thus, for example, if the Lung energy is weak then there may be a tendency for the Liver energy to be uncontrolled and to rise. This may manifest in problems like headaches or high blood pressure, for example. The problems may also occur in the opposite direction, which is seen as the natural 'controlling' function being rebelled against. For example, if the Spleen is overly damp, then this can have the problem of inhibiting the Liver's ability to move energy around the body.

The Cosmological Sequence

The third sequence that arises from the Five Element view, which has its roots not only in the Daoist nature view but also in Chinese numerology, places the Water Element at the root and thus at the most important point (see Figure 8).

As the Water Element is given the position at the root of the

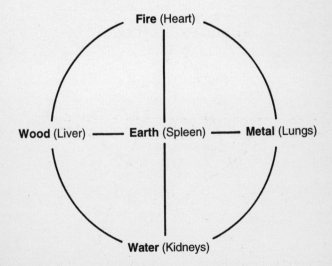

Figure 8. The Cosmological sequence: how the Five Elements mirror the Chinese view of the human body

sequence, this points to the importance in Chinese medicine of the Kidneys. The Kidneys are viewed as the root of the Yin and Yang energy in the body, and by implication, all the other organs. The Spleen, at the centre, is seen as the origin of Qi in the body and as such the focus of support of all the other organs.

The Five Element view is important from the perspective of demonstrating the way in which the Chinese system of medicine has built on the Daoist view of balance, process and harmony in the natural world. Some practitioners will approach their understanding of a patient's difficulties from the perspective of the Five Elements and build their interventions according to these principles. Other practitioners will take the basic Yin and Yang perspective and build up their understanding of the patient's difficulties by elaborating on ideas of excess and deficient energy patterns. It is this latter approach – reflecting the more dominant practices in China today – that will form the basis for outlining Chinese medicine principles throughout the rest of this book. However, readers interested in finding out more about the Five Element approach may care to explore some of the references given in bibliography.

SUMMARY

In the above sections you have been introduced to some of the basic ideas and principles that lie behind the practice of Chinese medicine. For the average Westerner these ideas do not sit comfortably with the view of the world that we have become accustomed to, but allowing the principles to germinate and take seed over time will pay handsome dividends. The Chinese system offers a way of looking at the world in general and our health patterns in particular in a uniquely holistic and comprehensive manner. It is important to understand that the practice of Chinese medicine, in whatever form it takes, has a history and set of principles as rich and as rigorous as those we hold so dear in Western society.

Do I Understand Yin and Yang?

The object of this exercise – which you should not take too seriously – is to see if you have really grasped the concept of Yin and Yang, which is so central to Chinese philosophy in general and to Chinese medicine in particular.

Below there is a list of twenty-five objects, situations, ideas and so on. For each one in turn decide whether it represents something that is predominately Yin or predominately Yang. Secondly, for each one, suggest how you might change it to represent the other quality – so, if you think the original is basically Yin, how would you change it to make it basically Yang and so on.

Here's an example to illustrate the process:

A cup of hot tea: This is predominately Yang in nature. Leave it to cool to room temperature for half an hour and it would become predominately Yin in nature.

Remember, in every situation Yin and Yang co-exist, it is just that there is a relative balance one way or the other. Also, Yin and Yang are continually interacting and in the process one will contain the other and transform into it. Ultimately, there are no absolute right or wrong answers in this exercise. Compare your answers to mine in the Appendix, but don't feel you necessarily have to agree with my analysis all the time.

There follows a list of twenty-five exemplars. In each case decide on the dominant Yin or Yang and how the one might transform into the other.

1. A rowdy school classroom.
2. A parked car.
3. A block of ice.
4. A thumping migraine headache.
5. An incomplete jigsaw puzzle.
6. A golfer lining up a putt.
7. A bout of diarrhoea.
8. An aeroplane taking off.
9. A politician delivering a speech.
10. A hard boiled egg.
11. A raw egg.
12. A CD of a heavy metal rock band.
13. A Mozart piano sonata being played.
14. A runner at the end of a marathon.
15. A coin.
16. A game of chess.
17. A packet of sherbet dip.
18. A car that has run out of petrol.
19. A book.
20. Someone performing a Taiqi exercise.

21. A baby with colic.
22. A hot summer's day.
23. A yawn.
24. A video of an aerobics exercise.
25. Your thought processes at this minute.

2

The Basic Substances

A S HAS BEEN pointed out, the conventional Western view of the human body emphasizes the physical structures and components that interact in a very subtle and complex manner. Anatomy and physiology map these structures from the largest – bones, muscles, skin and so on, to the smallest – cells and their components. This structural map forms the basis of the cause and effect model that dominates Western medical practice.

The Chinese model is very different. Here, we are looking at the components of process rather than of structure (see Chapter 4). The human body is first and foremost an energy system in which various substances interact with each other to create the physical organism. These basic substances, which range from the material to the immaterial, are Qi, Jing, Blood, Body Fluids and Shen.

Although we will be looking at each in turn, it is important always to remember that none can be considered as separate from the rest and that in the Chinese model there is a continuous dynamic interaction between them.

For each of the substances in turn we will consider:

- origin
- types
- functions
- disharmonies

QI

There is nothing more fundamental to Chinese medicine than understanding the concept of Qi (pronounced: 'Chee'; often written as Chi). Qi has variously been translated as 'energy', 'vital energy',

17

'life force' and so on, but the concept is impossible to capture fully in one English word or phrase. Everything in the universe is composed of Qi, yet it is neither seen as some fundamental particle or substance, nor as mere energy. Ted Kaptchuk is a well-respected Western practitioner of Chinese medicine who has written extensively for Western audiences. He perhaps captures best the essence of Qi when he describes it as 'matter on the verge of becoming energy, or energy at the point of materialising'.[1] As the Chinese say, 'when Qi gathers, so the physical body is formed; when Qi disperses, so the body dies'. Ultimately, it is probably wise not to debate endlessly what Qi is, rather it is best to try and understand Qi by being aware of what it does.

Origin and Types of Qi

This can best be illustrated by Figure 9.

The *Original Qi (Yuan Qi)* is also known as *Pre-Natal* or *Before Heaven Qi* and is inherited from our parents at conception.

There are two main sources of *Post-Natal* or *After Heaven Qi*, which are derived from the Qi in the world we live in. *Gu Qi* is derived from the food we eat and the main organ associated with this process is the Spleen. *Kong Qi* is derived from the air that we breathe and the main organ associated with this process is the Lung.

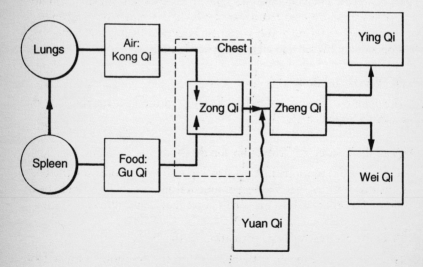

Figure 9. The origin of Qi

Gu Qi and *Kong Qi* mix together to form *Gathering Qi (Zong Qi)*, sometimes known as *Qi of the Chest*.

Finally, *Zong Qi* is catalyzed by the action of the *Yuan Qi* to form *Normal* or *Upright Qi (Zheng Qi)*, which becomes the Qi that circulates through the Channels and the Organs of the body.

Zheng Qi forms the basis of *Nutritive Qi (Ying Qi)*, which is essential in the process of nourishing all the tissues of the body. It also forms the basis of *Defensive Qi (Wei Qi)*, which circulates on the outside of the body and protects it from external factors that might cause disharmony and illness.

When *Zheng Qi* flows through each of the various internal organs of the body, the Qi functions with respect to the characteristics of that organ. Thus, for example, the activity of Liver Qi will be different from that of Lung Qi, but they are both manifestations of *Zheng Qi*. This is called *Organ Qi (Zangfu Zhi Qi)*. Similarly, when *Zheng Qi* flows through the Channels or Meridians of the body it is called *Meridian Qi (Jing Luo Zhi Qi)*.

Functions of Qi

There are five main functions of Qi in the body.

Qi Is the Source of Body Activity and Movement

Every aspect of movement in the body, both voluntary and involuntary, is a manifestation of the flow of Qi. Qi is constantly ascending, descending, entering and leaving the body and health and well-being is dependent on this continuous dynamic activity.

Qi Warms the Body

The maintenance of normal body temperature is a function of the warming action of Qi.

Qi Is the Source of Protection for the Body

As previously mentioned, Wei Qi is responsible for protecting the body from invasion by external environmental factors such as cold, heat, damp and other pathogenic factors that may cause illness.

Qi Is the Source of Transformation in the Body

The action of Qi in the body is crucial in the transformation of food and air into other vital substances, such as Qi itself, Blood and Body Fluids.

Qi Governs Retention and Containment

Healthy and strong Qi is vital in holding the various organs, vessels and tissues of the body in their correct place, hence facilitating their correct functioning. This would be analogous to the manner in which the correct pressure is needed in a tyre to bind it to the wheel and to facilitate the movement of the vehicle.

Disharmonies of Qi

There are generally four characteristic types of Qi disharmony.

Deficient Qi (Qi Xu)

In this instance there will be insufficient Qi to carry out adequately the various functions. Thus, for example, in older people a deficiency of Qi resulting from ageing can lead to chronic cold because the Qi is not performing its warming function adequately.

Sinking Qi (Qi Xian)

If the Qi is very deficient then it may no longer adequately perform its holding function and it may sink. This is most obviously seen in conditions such as organ prolapse.

Stagnant Qi (Qi Zhi)

If normal Qi flow is impaired for any reason, this can lead to sluggish flow or blockages. This would be analogous to a river that silts up. If not cleared, the water can become stagnant, putrid and incapable of sustaining life. A simple bump on the arm will cause localized swelling and pain because of the stagnation of Qi in the meridians. Stagnation can also affect internal organs leading to more serious disharmonies.

Rebellious Qi (Qi Ni)

In this instance, the Qi flows in the wrong direction. For example, Stomach Qi is characteristically considered to flow downwards, carrying food to the intestines. If the Stomach Qi 'rebels', it will move upwards, leading to problems such as hiccups, nausea and in extreme cases, vomiting.

JING

Jing, which is usually translated as Essence, is another somewhat difficult concept to understand in Chinese medicine. Jing can be considered the underpinning of all aspects of organic life. If Jing is plentiful there will be a strong life force and the organism will be healthy and radiant, whereas when Jing is lacking the life force will be weak and the organism will be susceptible to disease and disorders. It is perhaps useful to distinguish Jing from Qi by considering the notion of movement. As was shown above, Qi is responsible for the on-going day-to-day movements in the body, whereas Jing can be considered to be associated with slow developmental change that characterizes the organism's growth from a foetus through life and ultimately to old age and death.

Origins and Types of Jing

Before Heaven or *Congenital Jing* (*Xian Tian Zhi Jing*) is formed by the coming together of the sexual energies of the man and the woman in the act of conception. Thus, this *Congenital Jing* forms the basis for antenatal growth in the womb and nourishes the developing embryo and foetus. The quantity and quality of any individual's *Congenital Jing* is fixed and determines the constitution and characteristics of the person that they will take through life.

After Heaven or *Post-Natal Jing* (*Hou Tian Zhi Jing*) is the Jing that is obtained from ingested foods and fluids through the action of the Spleen and the Stomach. This *Post-Natal Jing* serves to supplement *Congenital Jing* and together they constitute the overall Jing of the organism.

Chinese medicine closely associates Jing with the function of the Kidneys and *Kidney Jing* represents a further distinction arising from both *Before Heaven* and *After Heaven Jing*. It will be sufficient for our discussion here to recognize that *Kidney Jing* promotes the transformation of Kidney Yin into Kidney Qi under the warming influence of Kidney Yang.

Functions of Jing

Jing Governs Growth, Reproduction and Development

Jing is seen as crucial to the development of the individual through life. In children it is responsible for the growth of bones, teeth and hair. It also promotes brain development and sexual maturation. In adulthood, Jing forms the basis of reproduction. Fertility in both the male and the female is dependent upon strong Kidney Jing.

Jing Promotes Kidney Qi

As pointed out above, the connection between Jing and the Kidneys is very strong. Kidney Qi is especially important as it is seen as the root of all the Qi in the body. Thus, if Kidney Qi is in any way deficient or weak then this will lead to a deficiency and weakness of the Qi of the whole body.

Jing Produces Marrow

In Chinese medicine the concept of Marrow goes beyond the Western notion of bone marrow to include the fundamental make-up of the spinal cord and the brain. Since Jing is responsible for the production of Marrow, there can be serious consequences if this process is weak.

Jing Forms the Basis of Our Constitution

The strength of our Jing determines our basic constitutional strength. Thus, the Jing works in concert with the Wei Qi to help protect the body from external factors. If Jing is weak the individual may be chronically prone to infection and illness.

Disharmonies of Jing

Jing disharmonies tend to relate directly to the functions outlined above.

Developmental Disorders

Any developmental disorder such as learning difficulties and physical disabilities in children is due to a deficiency of Jing. In later life, as Jing diminishes then physical deterioration occurs, commonly seen with deafness, greying and balding as well as general frailty and senility.

Kidney-related Disorders

Because of Jing's close association with the Kidneys, any deficiency can lead to Kidney-related problems such as impotence, low back pain and tinnitus.

Marrow-related Disorders

If Jing is weak then brain dysfunctions such as poor memory, poor concentration and dizziness can occur.

Constitutional Weakness

This can lead to a chronic tendency to external disease patterns and allergies that the individual will find very difficult to shake off.

BLOOD

The Western reader who is still having difficulty understanding the concepts of Qi and Jing will not find things getting any easier when discussing the significance of Blood in Chinese medicine.

Blood in Chinese medicine is not the same substance that is recognized as blood in Western medicine (we will use the upper case letter 'B' when referring to the Chinese use of the term, and the lower case letter 'b' when referring to the Western use of the term).

Chinese medicine sees Blood as a very material and fluid manifestation of Qi. In considering Blood we will slightly alter the focus of our discussion, looking at:

- origin of Blood
- functions of Blood
- inter-relationships with Blood
- disharmonies of Blood

Origin of Blood

It is thought there are two ways in which Blood is produced for use throughout the body.

Transformation of Food

This source of Blood is shown in Figure 10.

The Spleen extracts Gu Qi from the food ingested into the Stomach and this is sent upwards to the chest area. The Jing Qi begins the process of transformation into Blood and the Gu Qi is then sent from the Lungs to the Heart where the Yuan Qi facilitates the further transformation into Blood.

The Action of Marrow

This aspect of Blood production can be summarized in Figure 11.

In this instance, the Jing that is stored in the Kidneys produces Marrow. This in turn produces bone-marrow, which further contributes to the manufacture of Blood.

Thus, as can be seen, in Chinese medicine, the Spleen, Stomach, Lungs, Heart and Kidneys all have an important role to play in the development of Blood.

Functions of Blood

It is thought there are three functions of Blood in the body.

Blood Nourishes the Body

Probably the most important function of Blood is that by circulating continuously throughout the body it carries nourishment with it to all

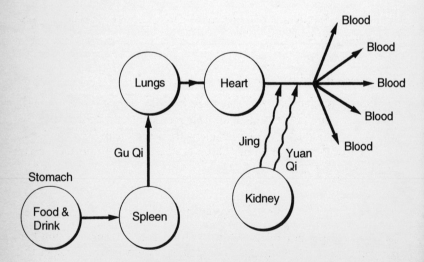

Figure 10. How Blood is manufactured from food

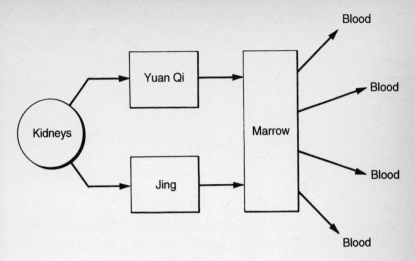

Figure 11. How Blood is produced via the action of Marrow in the body

the organs, muscles, tendons and so on. Remember that in Chinese medicine, Blood is seen as an aspect of Qi and as such it helps carry the nutritive aspects of Qi.

Blood Moistens the Body

Being a fluid, Blood has an important role in moistening and lubricating throughout the body.

Blood Aids the Mind (Shen)

Chinese medicine sees the Blood as helping to anchor the Mind, allowing for the development of clear and stable thought processes. When an individual is Blood-deficient then there can be a tendency towards irritability and anxiety because the Blood is not adequately anchoring the Mind.

Interrelationships with Blood

Blood has important relationships with all the Yin organs (Zang) of the body. This will be discussed in greater detail when we look at the function of the various organs in Chapter 4.

It is, however, worth saying a little more about the intimate interdependency between the Blood and Qi. Blood is an aspect of Qi. Qi can be considered Yang with respect to Blood since it is more ethereal and by implication, Blood is considered Yin with respect to Qi since it is more tangible. This close relationship can be seen in the following ways:

- Qi produces Blood.
- Qi moves Blood around the body.
- Qi holds the Blood in the blood vessels.
- Blood nourishes Qi.

The Chinese sum up this relationship between Qi and Blood by stating that 'Qi is the commander of Blood and Blood is the mother of Qi.'

Disharmonies of Blood

There are considered to be three main types of Blood disharmony.

Deficient Blood (Xue Xu)

If Blood is deficient this usually relates to the Spleen's inability to move Gu Qi for Blood production. Typically, this can lead to pale complexion, dry skin and dizziness on occasions.

Stagnant Blood (Xue Yu)

If Qi is weak or stagnant then it may fail to move the Blood adequately leading to stagnation of Blood. Typically, this will lead to sharp and often intense pain. There may also be the development of tumours.

Heat in the Blood

This usually results from internal heat generated by the disharmony of another organ – usually the Liver. This can lead to skin conditions and mental/emotional problems, among other disharmonies.

BODY FLUIDS

Body Fluids (Jin Ye) are considered to be the organic liquids that moisten and lubricate the body in addition to Blood, which is considered separately because of its importance in Chinese medicine.

Origin and Types of Body Fluids

Figure 12 illustrates the rather complex cycle of origin and transformation of Body Fluids.

Body Fluids originate in the process whereby the Spleen and Stomach function on ingested food and drink. In Chinese medicine an important function of the Spleen is to separate 'pure' from 'impure' fluids that are taken in food. The 'pure' fluids are sent upwards to the Lungs where they are further separated into 'light' fluids and 'dense' fluids. The 'light' fluids are dispersed by the Lungs to nourish and moisten the skin and the muscles of the body, while the 'dense' fluids are sent downwards to the Kidneys. The warming action of Kidney Yang further separates the 'dense' fluids sending the refined fluid back up to moisten the Lungs,

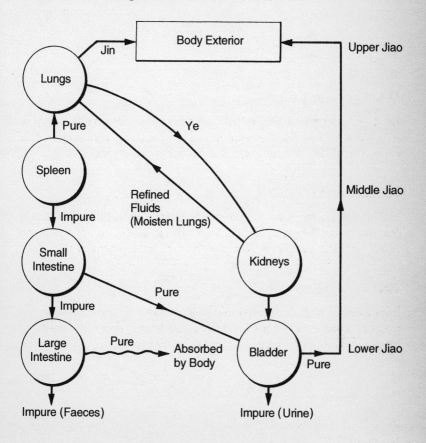

Figure 12. The production of Body Fluids

while the impure fluids go from the Kidney to the Bladder where they are excreted as urine.

In addition to this process, the 'impure' fluids from the Spleen are sent down to the Small Intestine, which further discriminates between purer fluids – sent to the Bladder and the most impure, which is sent to the Large Intestine for eventual excretion as faeces, although even then, some more pure distillate may be re-absorbed into the body. The final part of the Body Fluid cycle involves yet a further separation in the Bladder where the 'pure' is sent back up the body through the action of the San Jiao or Triple Warmer. The 'impure' is excreted as urine.

As is obvious, the production and circulation of Body Fluids is a subtle and complex process in Chinese medicine. At all stages there is a continuous process of separation and re-cycling in order to ensure that the maximum quantity of beneficial fluid is extracted and used by the body.

Essentially there are two types of Body Fluids.

Light Fluids (Jin)

The Jin fluids are light and watery and tend to be seen as circulating with the Wei Qi around the skin and the muscles on the exterior of the body. Their movement is controlled by the Lungs.

Dense Fluids (Ye)

The Ye fluids are much heavier and thicker. They are seen as circulating throughout the interior of the body with the Ying Qi under the influence of the Spleen and the Kidneys.

Function of Body Fluids

The function of all body fluids is basically to moisten and nourish the body.

The Jin fluids perform this function for the skin, the muscles and the hair. They can appear as fluids that flow directly from the body such as sweat, tears and saliva.

The Ye fluids perform this function for the joints and the brain.

Body Fluids, Qi and Blood

As should be becoming increasingly evident, in Chinese medicine we cannot think of any one of the vital substances existing functionally on its own. Their mutual functions continually interact and interrelate and this is well illustrated in thinking about Qi, Blood and the Body Fluids.

Qi is crucial in the production and the transportation of Body Fluids and it is responsible for holding the fluids in place. Conversely, if Body Fluids become deficient, then this can damage Qi, thus Body Fluids are essential for maintaining healthy Qi.

Body Fluids and Blood nourish each other, and Body Fluids are essential to maintain Blood at a consistency that will not stagnate, causing illness.

Disorders of Body Fluids

Essentially, there are two types of disorder that can arise with Body Fluids.

Deficient Body Fluids

This can lead to a whole range of problems arising from the lack of nourishing and moistening function. For example, deficient fluids in the Intestines can lead to constipation.

Accumulation of Fluids

If fluids accumulate this can lead to problems of Dampness and Phlegm in Chinese medicine. For example, if the Spleen is damaged by poor diet, this can lead to dampness that may manifest itself as lethargy and a feeling of heaviness in the lower abdomen.

SHEN

The last basic substance that we will briefly discuss is the Shen, which can be translated as the Mind or the Spirit of the individual. Mind is perhaps the most appropriate term to use, as Chinese philosophy distinguishes between several aspects of spirit, a discussion of which goes beyond the scope of this book.

However, we should not think of the Shen as simply the mind that thinks, memorizes and carries out logical processing. Hence, Shen is not human consciousness as such, but we can say that the existence of human consciousness is evidence of the action and presence of the Shen.

It is perhaps best to consider Shen in terms of its relationship with Qi and Jing.

Jing, Qi and Shen are referred to collectively in Chinese medicine as the 'Three Treasures' and are believed to be the essential components of the life of the individual.

- Jing is the densest component and is responsible for the developmental processes of the body.
- Qi is the next stage, responsible for the more immediate animate life of the body.
- Shen is the most refined level responsible for human consciousness.

When the Three Treasures are in harmony the individual will be radiant with life; physically fit, mentally sharp and alert. The driving force of the Shen suggests the personality of the individual.

Disharmonies of Shen

A minor Shen disturbance may present as slow and muddled thinking, anxiety or insomnia. In extreme instances, a Shen disharmony can produce a serious personality disorder, psychiatric disturbances and even unconsciousness.

SUMMARY

This chapter has introduced you at some length to the basic substances of Chinese medicine. As will be apparent, it presents as a very different picture to the Western tradition, but no less subtle and comprehensive for that.

It may be useful to summarize the various origins and functions of the fundamental substances in tabular form (see opposite).

A good rule of thumb to help you ease into these ideas is not to get caught up in trying to see Qi, Jing, Blood, Body Fluids and Shen as 'things' that make up the human being. Rather, continue to recognize that above all, process is being described by these ideas and that these basic substances exist in a constant dynamic equilibrium – they are the 'dance of life' in Chinese medicine!

The Basic Substances

	Origins	Functions
Qi	Before Heaven – parents After Heaven – food/air	movement and activity; warming; transformation; protection; containment
Jing	Before Heaven – parents After Heaven – ingested foods	growth, reproduction, development; promotes Kidney Qi; produces Marrow; constitutional basis
Blood	transformation of food; action of Marrow	nourishes; moistens; aids Shen
Body Fluids	distilled from ingested foods	moistens; nourishes via: Jin: light fluids Ye: dense fluids
Shen	manifestation of consciousness	keeps mind sharp and alert

Figure 12a. A summary table of the basic substances

3

The Meridian System

T HE AIM OF this chapter is to try and bring some clarity and logic to the understanding of the Energy distribution system of Chinese medicine and relate it to the overall discussion of Chinese medicine so far.

The term 'meridian' has been chosen to describe the overall system, but very often the meridians themselves will be described as 'channels' or even 'vessels' referring to specific pathways in the body. The choice is often one of personal preference, but the terms 'channels' and 'vessels' do tend to suggest the ideas of carrying, holding and transporting whereas 'meridian' is a more neutral term functionally.

WHAT ARE THE CHANNELS?

It will have been clear from the discussion in Chapter 2 on the basic substances that there must be a way in which these substances permeate the whole body. Chinese medicine describes a complex system of channels and their connecting vessels as the distribution system that carries Qi, Blood and the Body Fluids around the body.

It is tempting to think of the channels in the same way as we think of the system of blood vessels – arteries, veins, capillaries – that carry blood around the body. This is both a useful and a misleading analogy. It is useful to the extent that the channel system is indeed responsible for the distribution of the basic substances through the body, but it can be misleading in as much as conventional anatomy and physiology would not be able to identify these pathways in a physical sense in the way that blood vessels can be identified.

It should be remembered that Chinese medicine operates very much at a subtle energy level. Qi, Blood, Jing and Shen are essentially energetic properties that continually oscillate around the cusp of the physical and the energetic. The effects of the processes that they drive will manifest themselves in the physical body with all its strengths, weaknesses, idiosyncrasies and disharmonies, but they themselves remain essentially energetic in nature. Thus, it is perhaps more useful to consider the meridian system as an energetic distribution network that in itself tends towards an energetic manifestation. In much the same way that we try to understand Qi by its effects, similarly, the meridian system can best be understood as process rather than structure.

A useful analogy that is often used in Chinese medicine to describe Qi flow is that of a river. A river has a source and it follows its course ultimately towards the sea. As it flows it will vary from shallow to deep, quick flowing to slow flowing, while following the most 'natural' path.

Chinese philosophy believes that Qi permeates everything in the universe – there is nothing that is not a manifestation of Qi. Thus, Qi must permeate every microcosm of the human body, but there will be varying concentrations of Qi. It is perhaps useful to consider the meridian system as representing areas of high Qi concentration. Thus, as you move away from any given channel you do not suddenly reach an 'edge' – it is more a matter of moving from areas of high Qi concentration to ones of lower Qi concentration. This is similar to the way in which, as you move away from the centre of a river, the water becomes progressively more shallow and even when you move beyond the obvious physical boundary of the river there is still moisture contained within the soil.

Figure 13 tries to give a sense of what is being described.

Thus, we have the picture of the body being permeated by an energy system that concentrates around high energy density areas, which are termed channels. This energy is in constant dynamic movement in quite specific ways, as will be described later, driving the myriad of processes that manifest themselves as that physical organism. If anything occurs to weaken or block this energy flow in any way, then the result will be an energetic imbalance that in turn will manifest itself in the physical organism as disease or illness.

WHAT ARE ACUPUNCTURE POINTS?

The other feature that is always obvious on a meridian chart of the human body is the fact that the individual channels have specific points marked upon them. Some channels appear to have a lot, some

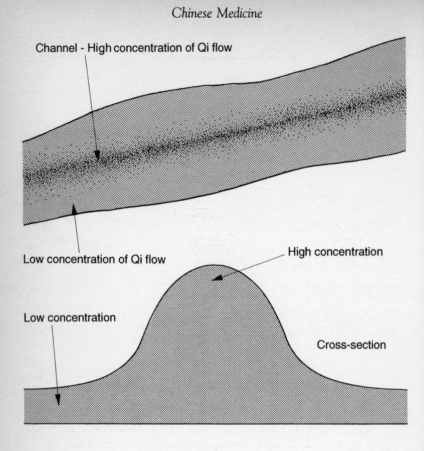

Channel - High concentration of Qi flow

Low concentration of Qi flow

High concentration

Low concentration

Cross-section

Figure 13. Qi flow in the body

have less, some points appear grouped close together and others appear more discrete. These are, of course, what are commonly described as acupuncture points, but how do they relate to this dynamic energy system that we have been describing above?

It would appear that along many of the channels there are what could be best described as 'access points'. Going back again to the analogy of the river, consider how a whirlpool effect draws everything down into the heart of the river – it gives access to the depth of the river in effect. It is therefore perhaps useful to consider acupuncture points as 'energy vortices' that draw Qi into or out of the body's energy flow and that provide an access point whereby the Qi flow of the body can be directly influenced (see Figure 14).

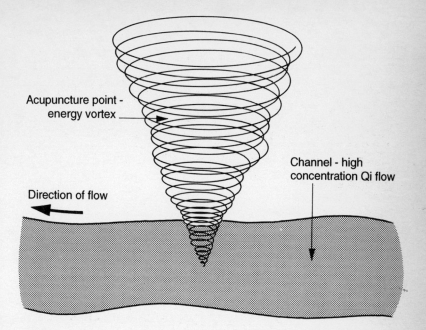

Acupuncture point - energy vortex

Channel - high concentration Qi flow

Direction of flow

Figure 14. An acupuncture point

Thus, simple pressure on a specific 'energy vortex' will produce changes in the energy system with consequent physical effects. This would, of course, be the basis for simple acupressure treatment. It is likely that we use instinctively such techniques when suffering from a minor disharmony. For example, rubbing the temple area on the side of our head when suffering a headache – this would stimulate the 'energy vortex' or acupuncture point known as Taiyang. Acupuncture simply takes this a stage further. The fine needles would be inserted into the patient's energy system at a series of appropriately selected vortices, or acupuncture points. The effect of the needling would be to cause changes in the pattern of the patient's energy system resulting in, hopefully, beneficial changes taking place at the physical level. It is likely that the practitioner's own energy system is also a factor in the process, the needle in effect becoming an extension of that energy system.

Hopefully, by now the reader will have a more dynamic view of the body's energy system that will help in understanding the concept of the meridian system as a form of 'energy anatomy'. The whole issue of energy anatomy will be revisited in a more speculative manner in Chapter 8.

THE MERIDIAN SYSTEM IN CHINESE MEDICINE

Discussion will be limited to describing the channels in terms of their relationships and their functions – any reader wishing to study the system in more detail should refer to the Bibliography. Figure 15 shows the system.

Taking the anatomical diagram on face value it would appear that the meridian system is made up of a series of independent channels that run on the surface of the body – nothing could be further from the truth.

The channels can be classified into various types.

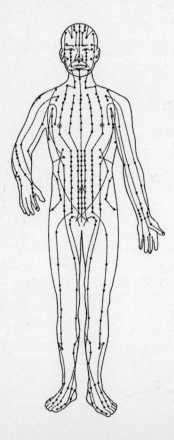

Figure 15. The basic meridian systems in the body

The Twelve Regular Channels (Jing)

These twelve regular channels correspond to the five Yin organs, the six Yang organs and the Pericardium, which is functionally considered a Yin organ in Chinese medicine.

There are three Yin organs and three Yang organs relating to both the arm and the leg. Each Yin organ is paired with its corresponding Yang organ. These Yin/Yang correspondences are as follows:

Yin Organ	Yang Organ
Lung	Large Intestine
Heart	Small Intestine
Pericardium	San Jiao
Liver	Gall Bladder
Kidney	Bladder
Spleen	Stomach

The San Jiao is an organ in Chinese medicine that has no anatomical counterpart in Western medicine. This will be discussed in greater detail in Chapter 4.

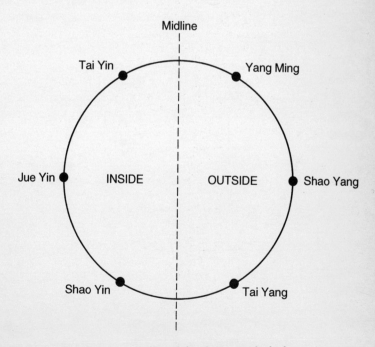

Figure 16. Channel distribution in the limbs

If we consider a cross-section of a limb, the relative positions of the channels are as shown in Figure 16.

There are six paired Yin channels and six paired Yang channels (three of each on the arm and the leg respectively). Thus we have:

Arm Tai Yin Channel:	Lung
Leg Tai Yin Channel:	Spleen
Arm Shao Yin Channel:	Heart
Leg Shao Yin Channel:	Kidney
Arm Jue Yin Channel:	Pericardium
Leg Jue Yin Channel:	Liver
Arm Yang Ming Channel:	Large Intestine
Leg Yang Ming Channel:	Stomach
Arm Tai Yang Channel:	Small Intestine
Leg Tai Yang Channel:	Bladder
Arm Shao Yang Channel:	San Jiao
Leg Shao Yang Channel:	Gall Bladder

Qi Flow Circulation in the Twelve Regular Channels

Qi flows from the chest area along the three arm Yin channels (Lu; Per; He) to the hands. There they connect with the three paired arm Yang channels (LI; SJ; SI) and flow upwards to the head. In the head they connect with their three corresponding leg Yang channels (St; GB; Bl) and flow down the body to the feet. In the feet they connect with their corresponding leg Yin channel (Sp; Liv; Kid) and flow up again to the chest to complete the cycle of Qi circulation.

Although Qi is continuously circulating through the twelve regular channels at all times, there are recognized times when the Qi and Blood flow is at its maximum in each given channel. Thus, the flow in relation to the daily cycle of maximum in each channel is as follows:

Lung (3am–5am) → Large Intestine (5am–7am) → Stomach (7am–9am) → Spleen (9am–11am) → Heart (11am–1pm) → Small Intestine (1pm–3pm) → Bladder (3pm–5pm) → Kidney (5pm–7pm) → Pericardium (7pm–9pm) → San Jiao (9pm–11pm) → Gall Bladder (11pm–1am) → Liver (1am–3am)

This information can be of great assistance to the practitioner in considering diagnosis and treatment strategies.

Channel Functions

The channels have the function of being the energetic unification structures of the whole body. They connect the interior with the exterior and are the pathways and concentrations of Qi and Blood flow throughout the body. They exercise the apparently contradictory functions of carrying the protective Wei Qi throughout the body, but they are also the route through which external pathogenic factors can invade the body, initially the exterior, but also to the interior.

Also, importantly, the channels provide the practitioner with the 'entry points' to access the Qi flow with acupuncture.

Channel Communication

The arm and leg channels of the same name are considered to 'communicate' with each other in Chinese medicine. Thus, problems in a given channel or organ can be treated by using points on the communication partner. For example, a disharmony in the Lungs can be treated by using points on the Spleen channel – they are both Tai Yin channels.

Each channel also relates to its corresponding organ. This is an example of an exterior/interior communication. Also, each channel will relate to its paired Yin or Yang organ. Let's illustrate this with a couple of examples.

1. If there is a problem on the Large Intestine channel this can be treated by points on the Large Intestine channel and also by points on the Lung channel (paired Yin of Large Intestine).
2. If the Kidneys have a problem, this can be treated by points on the Kidney channel and also by points on the Bladder channel (paired Yang of the Kidneys).

Regular Channel Disharmonies

It should be borne in mind that when a disharmony occurs in a given organ, the problem can spill over into related organs through the channel system.

For example, someone who follows an excessively 'cold' diet of, say, salads, cold and raw foods, fruit and iced drinks, can cause the Stomach to become Qi deficient. This can affect the Yang energy of the Spleen (paired organ) resulting in the Spleen Qi being unable to rise. Consequently, the Spleen energy will fall, leading to problems such as diarrhoea. The connection of the Stomach with the Large Intestine (Yang Ming channels) will also exacerbate the disharmony.

The Eight Extraordinary Channels

These eight channels do not have the direct linkage to the major Zangfu organ system and only two of them have acupuncture points on them.

The eight extraordinary channels are:

Ren Mai	Conception vessel
Du Mai	Governing vessel
Chong Mai	Penetrating vessel
Dai Mai	Girdle vessel
Yin Wei Mai	Yin linking vessel
Yang Wei Mai	Yang linking vessel
Yin Qiao Mai	Yin heel vessel
Yang Qiao Mai	Yang heel vessel

The most important of these channels are the Du Mai and Ren Mai. They both have acupuncture points on them that are independent of the twelve regular channels. The other six are considered less important and they share points with points on the twelve regular channels.

Functions of the Extraordinary Channels

There are various specific functions that can be highlighted.

1. They act as reservoirs of Qi and Blood for the twelve regular channels, filling and emptying as required.
2. They circulate Jing around the body because they have a strong connection with the Kidneys.
3. They help circulate the defensive Wei Qi over the trunk of the body and as such they play an important role in maintaining health.
4. They provide further connections between the twelve regular channels.

The Divergent Channels

Each of the twelve regular channels has what is termed a divergent channel. They provide a connection from the Yin channels to their associated Zang organs and from the Yang channels to their associated Fu organs.

The Finer Network Channels (Luo)

Blood flow has major distribution vessels – arteries and veins – but there are also a myriad of tiny connecting capillaries that ensure blood flows to every corner of the body. In the same way, the meridian system is made up of a network of small connecting channels.

Fifteen Connecting Channels

These channels provide the connection between the Yin and Yang channel pairs, for example between the Heart and the Small Intestine channels.

Each of the twelve regular channels has a connecting channel, the Spleen channel has two and the Ren Mai and Du Mai have one each – making fifteen channels in total.

Minute/Superficial/Blood Channels

These are a myriad of tiny connecting channels that make up the total matrix of the meridian system.

CONCLUSION

A brief overview of the energy anatomy system of channels and acupuncture points, which are central to understanding how the practitioner of Chinese medicine begins to observe and understand the processes associated with Qi and Blood flow, has been given. The practitioner must be as knowledgeable about these networks as the Western doctor is about the anatomy and physiology of the physical body. Without that understanding successful intervention would be very difficult.

Experience Your Own Qi Flow

One of the main problems that people have with Chinese medicine is coming to terms with a system and a process that cannot be directly observed. We can easily experience our blood flow by pricking our finger, but experiencing our Qi flow is not so easy.

This is a simple Qigong exercise that may allow you to begin to experience the effects of Qi flow.

1. Sit comfortably with your feet resting flat on the floor and your back upright. Place your hands face up in your lap
2. Take two or three minutes just to relax.
3. Bring your arms to about chest height with the palms facing each other about 6 to 8 inches apart. The arms should be relaxed. Avoid having them straight out with the muscles tense. Imagine you are holding a soft flexible beach ball between your hands.

4. Breathe naturally, expanding your lower abdomen – the area known in Chinese medicine as the lower Dan Tien – on the inhalation. Imagine your Qi moving from this area about two finger breadths below your umbilicus. This point on the Ren channel is called Qihai, or 'sea of Qi'.
5. Imagine the Qi rising up the Ren channel and out along the Yin channels on the inside of the arm. In particular, pay attention to the Pericardium channel that runs right down the centre of the inside arm to end at the tip of the middle finger.
6. With each exhalation imagine the Qi flowing down the Pericardium channel to the palm of the hand. Focus on the Laogong point in the centre of the palm. This is Pericardium 8.
7. Begin to become aware of your experience at the Laogong points on the two opposite palms as you continue to relax and breathe easily. You may have a variety of experience – warmth, coolness, tingling, heaviness, a sense of attraction between the palms and so on. Just be aware of the feeling.
8. Play with the experience by bringing the two palms closer together and then pulling them apart. You may like to run the palm of one hand up the outside of the opposite arm from the thumb to the elbow. Keep it about an inch above the arm. Be aware if you experience any 'hot spots' as you go where Laogong seems to be making a connection with a point on the opposite arm. This may well be noticed at the point Hegu (on the fleshy mound between the thumb and the forefinger) or at the point Quchi, which is at the elbow.

As you do this simple exercise you will begin to experience the effect of Qi flow, whether as heat, cold or whatever. Remember, the sensation is not the Qi, it is the effect of Qi.

Think of this analogy. If electricity passes through a wire it will meet resistance. If the resistance rises the current flow will cause the wire to heat up. The heat in the wire is *not* the electricity, it is the *effect* of the electricity flow.

Think of your experience in this exercise in the same way. What you are experiencing is the effect of Qi flow. The point to emphasize is that there is no one sensation to be looking for. They can vary, but some form of warmth tends to be the most common.

If you practise Qigong exercises on a regular basis then your ability to become aware of your own Qi flow, and indeed that of other people, will develop markedly. You may wish to refer to some of the Qigong books in the Bibliography.

4

The Zangfu System

IN THIS CHAPTER we will look at a system that is of fundamental importance in understanding the way Chinese medicine sees the functioning of the human body. We will explore the basic ideas behind the Zangfu and then look in more detail at the features of this with respect to each of the Zangfu in turn.

PROCESS AND STRUCTURE

The first point that needs addressing is that of the difference between process and structure.

The Body Organs as Physical Structures

This idea seems so self-evident to the Western mind that we have to wonder why state it at all. It is important to state the obvious in order to emphasize just what a difference the non-obvious implies.

The gift that Western anatomy and physiology has given to the world is an immensely sophisticated view of the structures of the physical body. Among these structures the individual organs are emphasized in terms of their biology and function. Thus, for example, the heart is seen as a very complex and reliable pump that ensures a constant flow of blood around the whole body.

The Western approach to medicine has concerned itself, almost exclusively, with trying to understand how these structures function when normal and the ways in which this normal function can break down. Therapy then, has the goal of trying to restore the malfunctioning structure to good working order.

It is important to understand that there is absolutely nothing wrong with this way of seeing the body and, indeed, it has brought us some remarkable medical breakthroughs that would have been inconceivable a few decades ago.

We will, however, find this 'common sense' understanding stretched to the limit when we begin to look at the Chinese model. Indeed, a good rule of thumb to adopt when looking at the Chinese medicine approach is to leave our conventional wisdom to one side.

Experience dictates that if you try to combine the two systems then the conceptual problems that follow only hinder understanding.

The Body Organs as Processes

In Chinese medicine the first thing that will become obvious is that very little is said about organs as structures, but an awful lot is said about how an organ system is part of the overall dynamic energy process of the human body.

In every instance the emphasis will be on how the organs ensure the constant ebb and flow of the fundamental substances of the body. Illness is seen as a process disharmony that needs alleviating, not a 'machinery breakdown' that requires to be fixed.

Now this distinction may seem like semantic juggling, but hopefully the full significance will emerge as we explore the process function of each of the organ systems in turn.

SO, WHAT ARE THE ZANGFU ANYWAY?

The term Zangfu can be considered as the collective name for the series of Yin and Yang organ systems that are identified in Chinese medicine. These systems can be described as follows.

The Yin Organs – the Zang

In the theory of Chinese medicine, the Zang consist of the five solid (Yin) organs. These are:

- Spleen
- Heart
- Lungs
- Liver
- Kidneys

There is also considered to be a sixth Yin Zang, namely the Pericardium. It has its own Qi meridian, but to all intents and purposes its function is closely associated with the Heart.

In general, Chinese medicine considers the Zang to be deeper in the body and to be concerned with the manufacture, storage and regulation of the fundamental substances.

The Yang Organs – the Fu

In the theory of Chinese medicine, the Fu consist of the six hollow (Yang) organs. These are:

- Small Intestine
- Large Intestine
- Gall Bladder
- Bladder
- Stomach
- San Jiao (sometimes called Triple Warmer or Triple Heater)

In general, Chinese medicine considers the Fu to be closer to the surface of the body and to have the functions of receiving, separating, distributing and excreting body substances. The Fu are not considered as storage organs, but organs where there is an ongoing movement and change.

The Fu give the first really interesting distinction between the Western view and the Chinese view regarding structure and process. The San Jiao is considered an organ in Chinese medicine because its processes can be identified, but at the same time there is obviously no anatomical structure that can be identified as the San Jiao. Once you are able to appreciate the concept of the San Jiao, then you can be confident that you are well on your way to getting to grips with the system of Chinese medicine.

The Extra Fu (or Extraordinary Fu)

In addition to the main breakdown into the Zangfu, the traditional Chinese medicine system also identifies a series of less important organs in terms of process. They are:

- Brain
- Uterus
- Marrow
- Bone

- Blood Vessels
- Gall Bladder (Note: the Gall Bladder is considered both a Fu and an Extra Fu – just to complicate the picture still further!)

It will now be useful in our discussion of the Zangfu to consider the functions and processes of each of the Zang and Fu in turn. With each of the descriptions of the Zangfu, there will be given simple examples of a common disharmony of that particular organ. This will be for illustrative purposes and will be elaborated upon when considering Zangfu disharmonies in more detail in subsequent chapters.

THE FUNCTIONS OF THE ZANG

The Heart

The Heart Governs the Blood

This function of the Heart is the closest to the conventional Western view. The Heart controls and regulates the flow of blood through the vessels of the body. This is essential to ensure a healthy supply of Blood to all the tissues of the body. A healthy functioning will result in an even warmth in the extremities of the body and a regular and even pulse. Impaired functioning may lead to cold extremities and abnormal pulse patterns and in serious cases, classic heart-related chest pains.

The Heart also has the function of transforming the Qi from food (Gu Qi) into Blood and a poor diet can be seen as impairing Heart function.

Heartbeat, which moves the blood, is aided by the Zong Qi of the chest, which also has a role in respiration of the Lungs.

The Heart Controls the Blood Vessels

The function of the Heart is reflected in the healthy functioning of the blood vessels. In Chinese medicine the vessels are seen as an extension of the Heart. Good function will lead to healthy circulation, while impaired functioning may lead to conditions such as hardening of the arteries.

The Heart Houses the Shen

As has been discussed in an earlier chapter, the concept of the Shen is a complex one in Chinese medicine and can have a variety of meanings. For our purposes here it is important to consider that the Shen represents the myriad of mental, psychological and spiritual faculties that constitute a central feature of the human condition. It is probably best described as the force that shapes our personalities. When the Heart has the Shen under control then we can use the attributes of our personality in a constructive and healthy fashion. If the Heart fails to house the Shen, then this can lead to a whole range of mental and psychological disorders. It is often said in Chinese medicine that the health of the Shen can be viewed in the eyes!

The Heart Manifests in the Complexion

Since it is the function of the Heart to ensure the smooth flow of Blood around the body and through the vessels, it is considered important to gauge the functioning of the Heart by looking at the complexion. When the Heart is healthy there will be a strong rosy and lustrous complexion, whereas if there is deficient Heart function then the complexion will be dull. If the function is impaired to the point of Blood stagnation then the complexion may be blue or purple in tinge.

The Heart Opens into the Tongue

It is often said in Chinese medicine that 'the tongue is the mirror of the Heart'. Although the condition of other organs can be gauged from the tongue, it is the Heart function that most readily manifests in the tongue – especially in the tip. If Heart Blood is deficient then the tongue will be pale and if there is a stagnation of Heart Blood, then the tongue will appear purple in colour.

The Heart Controls Sweat

In Chinese medicine, Blood and Body Fluids are seen as having a common origin and there is a continuous interchange between the two. Thus, if a patient is sweating in an abnormal way then consideration has to be given to the role that the Heart Blood has in this.

The Heart Maintains Joy

The emotion that is associated with the Heart in the Chinese system is joy. The extent to which a person manifests appropriate joy in their life will often reflect the health of their Heart function. As with everything in Chinese medicine, emotions are seen in balance and not as extremes. Thus, a tendency to over-express joyful emotions in an inappropriate manner can be seen as a disharmony just as much as an overly negative and pessimistic disposition.

The Spleen

The Spleen Governs Transportation and Transformation

In Chinese medicine, the Spleen is seen as the primary organ of digestion. The Spleen extracts the nutrients from food in the Stomach (Gu Qi), which form the basis of Qi and Blood and transports it to the Lungs and the Heart for transformation into Qi and Blood. A healthy Spleen will mean good appetite, digestion, energy and muscle tone. When the Spleen's function is impaired this will lead to fatigue, abdominal distension, poor digestion and diarrhoea. The Spleen also transforms and transports fluids throughout the body. When the Spleen is impaired this will lead to an accumulation of body fluids leading to internal damp. This may manifest as oedema, obesity and phlegm-related disorders.

The Spleen Contains the Blood

The Spleen has the function of ensuring that the Blood flow is controlled within the blood vessels. This is distinct from the Heart function, which ensures that the Blood flows, that is, it is 'pumped'. If Spleen function is impaired then this can result in Blood leakages that can manifest themselves as blood in the stools and urine or a tendency to bruise easily. Varicose veins may also be seen as a Spleen-related disorder.

The Spleen Dominates the Muscles and the Limbs

The Spleen has the function of transporting refined Qi throughout the body and this ensures that the muscles and the limbs have good tone and shape. If the Spleen Qi is deficient in any way, then the refined Qi will not adequately tonify the flesh resulting in fatigue, thin, weak and flabby muscles. In any condition where tiredness is present, then it will be important to work with the Spleen.

The Spleen Opens into the Mouth and Manifests Itself in the Lips

The mouth has a crucial role in preparing food for digestion and as such it is closely related to the Spleen in Chinese medicine. When the Spleen is healthy then the sense of taste will be sharp and the lips moist and rosy. If there is a Spleen disharmony then the sense of taste will be dulled and the lips will become pale and dry.

The Spleen Controls the Raising of the Qi

A general feature of Spleen function is that it has a lifting effect on the energy of the body from the midline. Thus, the Spleen will hold internal organs in place.

When there is a Spleen disharmony then this is likely to lead to conditions such as internal prolapse and an imbalance of normal function leading to conditions such as diarrhoea.

The Spleen Houses Thought

As a result of the raising function of the Spleen, it has the role of sending clear energy to the head and brain. This results in a clarity of thought that can give the sense of lightness and well-being. Thus the ability to think clearly and concentrate well is dependent on a healthy Spleen function.

When the Spleen is impaired there will be a deficiency of clear energy reaching the head, which can result in muzzy and at times, disordered thinking. This can lead to a form of psychological block, where it becomes difficult to make decisions and move on in any facet of life. A corollary of this is when someone is engaged in an excess of concentration and thinking (for example a student studying), then this can in turn damage the Spleen, leading to fatigue and lethargy.

The Kidneys

The Kidneys Store Jing and Dominate Reproduction, Growth and Development

As was pointed out before, Jing is the essence of life and this is stored in the Kidneys. This is, in part, inherited from our parents and, in part, refined essence extracted from food.

Jing determines our constitutional strength and is an essential component of every aspect of the body. It is particularly the basis of growth and development through childhood and also fundamental to normal sexual and reproductive functioning.

When Kidney Jing is impaired in any way – often for constitutional reasons – then this can lead to retarded growth, learning difficulties, infertility, sexual disorders and premature senility.

The Kidneys Produce Marrow, Fill Up the Brain, Dominate the Bones and Manufacture Blood

There is a set of connections between these apparently disparate issues that connects them all to the Kidneys. Kidney Jing is responsible for the production of Marrow. In Chinese medicine, Marrow is the essential element of bone, bone marrow, the spinal cord and brain structure. Thus, healthy Kidney Jing will result in strong bones and teeth and efficient brain function.

If Marrow production is impaired in any way then this may result in a whole variety of problems, including tinnitus, blurred vision, impaired thinking and aching low back. Marrow also has a role in manufacturing Blood, so impaired Kidney function can also lead to Blood deficiency.

The Kidneys Maintain the Gate of Vitality (Fire of Mingmen)

In Chinese medicine, the Mingmen Fire is the source of all heat in the body. The maintenance of this essential Fire represents the Yang aspect of Kidney function. If the Kidney Yang energy is deficient then this will affect the Mingmen Fire, possibly resulting in general coldness, lethargy, impaired sexual function and, by damaging the Spleen, it can also lead to poor digestion.

The Kidneys Govern Water

A central function of the Kidneys is to regulate the fluid balance in the body. As the Kidneys dominate the Lower Jiao, often called 'the drainage ditch', they can be seen as having the function of eliminating any waste water from the body.

When the Kidneys are functioning well they are able to send the clear fluids back to the Lungs and excrete the dirty fluids through the Bladder. If Kidney function is impaired then this can lead to a whole range of urinary problems.

The Kidneys Control the Reception of Qi

This function represents the harmonious relationship between the Kidneys and the Lungs. The Lungs descend Qi and the Kidneys have the function of holding the Qi down, thus facilitating the healthy breathing process.

If the Kidney function is impaired, then this can lead to the Qi rebelling upwards causing breathing difficulties and, in extreme cases, chronic asthma. Thus, in Chinese medicine, the role of the Kidneys in facilitating healthy breathing is very important.

The Kidneys Open into the Ear

The ears rely on Kidney Jing for nourishment, and if this is in any way lacking, then it can lead to tinnitus and deafness. As Jing diminishes with age, it is seen that older people often start to have problems with their hearing.

The Kidneys Manifest in the Hair

The hair also relies on Kidney Jing for nourishment. In normal functioning, the hair will be healthy and glossy. If, on the other hand, there is a deficiency, then this is liable to lead to dull, lifeless and brittle hair. It can also lead to premature greying and thinning.

The Kidneys House the Will and Control Fear

The connection between will power and the emotion of fear is seen in the Kidneys. The Kidneys are seen as the root of life and as such our sense of personal power and will to succeed in life is rooted in healthy Kidney functioning.

Consequently, poor Kidney functioning will lead to feelings of weakness and timidity – being unable to face the very demands of life itself.

The Lungs

The Lungs Govern Qi and Respiration

The most important function of the Lungs is both similar to, yet different from, the conventional Western view. The Lungs govern inhalation of pure Qi from the air, and the exhalation of impure Qi. The crucial difference lies in the Chinese medicine view that it is the Qi we get from the air that is important, not just the oxygen as such. When the Lungs are functioning well then the respiration pattern is smooth and regular.

The second aspect of governing Qi lies in the role that the Lungs take in the formation of the Qi we use in our bodies. The Spleen sends up the Qi extracted from food to the Lungs where it combines with the pure Qi inhaled in the air to form what is called Zong Qi, which is the aspect of Qi that ensures that the Lungs help to spread Qi to all parts of the body. If there is any imbalance in the Lungs, then this can lead to general symptoms of Qi deficiency affecting the whole body and causing general weakness and tiredness.

The Lungs Control Dispersion and Descending

The Lungs disperse defensive Qi (Wei Qi) and body fluids throughout the most superficial layers of the body. If the Lungs are healthy then this keeps the body at even temperature and also protects the body from invasion by external pathogenic factors such as Cold, Wind and Damp. If the Lung Qi is weak then the body is liable to be very susceptible to disease. Thus, for example, when we 'catch a cold' our Lung Qi is likely to be depleted thus allowing the cold to invade the body, and the organ that is most immediately affected is, of course, the Lungs. In terms of the body fluids, the Lungs control the healthy functioning of sweating and if abnormal sweating occurs, the Lungs are likely to be affected.

Chinese medicine describes the Lungs as the uppermost Zang in the body and as such it is said that the natural function of the Lungs is a descending one. The Lungs send the Qi down to the Kidneys (the lowest Zang) where it is 'held down'. This dynamic between the Lungs and the Kidneys is vital to healthy respiration. If the descending function is impaired then this may lead to chest problems including coughing, congestion and even asthma.

The Lungs also send down body fluids to the Kidneys where they are separated into pure and impure. Healthy Lungs will ensure healthy fluid metabolism, whereas an impaired Lung function will lead to swelling and oedema in the upper part of the body, mainly the face.

The Lungs Regulate the Water Passages of the Body

As discussed above, the Lungs have a role to play in ensuring that body fluids are dispersed healthily throughout the body. Impaired Lung function can lead to retention of urine.

The Lungs Control the Skin and the Hair

As has been pointed out, the Lungs have a vital role to play in ensuring that Qi and fluids flow smoothly and effectively in the outermost parts of the body. Thus, it is seen in Chinese medicine that the Lungs have a powerful influence over the skin and the sweat glands. If Lung function is impaired then this may lead to rough and dry skin. In Chinese medicine, skin conditions are always seen as being evidence of a Lung disharmony. It is interesting to note that Chinese medicine provides a strong basis for the observed connection between skin allergies and Lung allergies, for example asthma and eczema.

In terms of hair, the Lungs control the condition of general body hair. The hair on our head is seen as being related to Kidney function, as discussed before. The health of general body hair is closely related to the condition of the skin.

The Lungs Open into the Nose

The nose is seen as the opening of the Lungs and as such the condition of the Lungs will determine factors such as how clear the nose is and how acute our sense of smell is. Clearly, when Lung function is impaired then so are these factors.

The Lungs Bring Us a Sense of Connection to the World

The theory of Chinese medicine sees the Lungs as being responsible for the extent to which we make healthy and constructive connections with the world we live in. With healthy Lung function we are able to maintain structures in our dealing with others. Impaired Lung function can lead to a sense of alienation.

In particular, the emotion associated with the Lungs is grief. When we deal with loss and change in a healthy way our sense and experience of grief can be controlled and helpful. If the Lungs are impaired then we may find it very difficult to work through grief and cope with change.

The Liver

The Liver Stores Blood

A major function of the Liver is to regulate the amount of Blood in circulation. This will naturally vary depending upon the demands of physical activity. Thus, when the body needs increased Blood flow, the Liver will release Blood and when the body requires less Blood flow it is the role of the Liver to store the excess until it is needed again. In healthy Liver function the body will receive a good Blood supply and will be healthy, strong and flexible. If there is impaired Liver function then weakness and stiffness may ensue.

In women, because of this role in storing and releasing Blood, the Liver is closely associated with menstruation and many gynaecological problems are likely to be related to the Liver function.

The Liver Controls the Smooth Flow of Qi

This is by far one of the most important functions of the Liver. The free flow of Qi throughout the body is crucial to the health of all functions in the body and it is because of this that stagnant Liver Qi is often associated with many other disharmonies that may be observed. Clinically, it is probably the most common disharmony that a practitioner of Chinese medicine will see. Problems arising from stagnant Liver Qi will be discussed in greater detail later in this book.

This smoothing and flowing function of the Liver is also seen as relating to the harmonization of emotions. When there is emotional stagnation then problems such as anger and frustration can arise.

The Liver Controls the Tendons

In Chinese medicine, the concept of 'tendons' covers ligaments, tendons and the manner in which they interact with the muscles. Thus, the Liver is seen as being very important in terms of our capacity for movement and flexibility. The tendons' capacity to expand and contract effectively depends on the nourishment from Liver Blood, which in turn requires the smooth flow of Liver Qi.

The Liver Manifests in the Nails

Chinese medicine sees the nails as belonging to the tendons, hence the connection with the Liver. If Liver Blood is healthy then the nails will be strong and moist. If there is a problem with Liver Blood, then this is likely to lead to thin, brittle and pale nails.

The Liver Opens into the Eyes

The eyes require the nourishment of Liver Blood in order to see clearly. Thus, the condition and health of the eyes is seen as being dependent on the health of Liver function. When Liver Blood is deficient, then this may lead to a variety of eye disorders.

The Liver Exercises Control

In Chinese medicine, the Liver is seen as the Zang that helps us keep control of our life in all its facets. When the Liver is balanced and functioning well then we can exercise effective control over the events in our life and we respond to sudden changes in a considered and flexible manner. On the other hand, if the Liver function is in any way impaired there can be a tendency to become overcontrolling, rigid and inflexible, or to become undercontrolling, which may lead to outbursts of anger and irrational emotional reactions. Liver disharmonies are always present in any stress-related disorder.

The Pericardium

It is important to mention the first anomaly at this point. In traditional Chinese medicine the Pericardium is considered to be a Yin organ, but it is not considered to be one of the five major Zang organs. In practical terms, the Pericardium is closely allied to the Heart.

The Pericardium Protects the Heart

In Western medicine the Pericardium is seen as the protective outer covering of the Heart. This is mirrored in Chinese medicine, which sees the Pericardium as protecting the Heart from invasion by external pathogenic factors, such as high fever. The heat in such an instance would be contained by the Pericardium, thus protecting the major Yin organ, the Heart.

The Pericardium Guides Joys and Pleasures

This rather vague function of the Pericardium seems to relate to the Heart's association with the emotion of joy. It is important to realize that Chinese medicine would consider either too little or too much joy in one's life as an example of a disharmony. Thus, in its role as protecting the Heart the Pericardium seeks to guide us through life to experience joy and pleasure in a manner that is balanced.

In this section, we have gone through the functions of each of the Yin organs in some detail. It should now be becoming clearer why there is such an emphasis on process in Chinese medicine. When we look at some common disharmonies later in the book, it will be seen that the complexity of the Zangfu does not end here. Their functions interact with each other and the cocktail of influence that results makes Chinese medicine both frustrating and yet endlessly fascinating.

Before considering how this all fits together, we should take a brief look at the function of the Yang organs of the body – the Fu. For the purposes of this book the main focus will be upon the Zang organs, but an awareness of the Fu is important (see Bibliography).

THE FUNCTIONS OF THE FU

The Gall Bladder

The Gall Bladder Stores Bile

This is stored and excreted into the digestive tract to aid digestion.

The Gall Bladder Dominates Decision-Making

The theory of Chinese medicine sees the Gall Bladder as bestowing the capacity to make judgements. Gall Bladder impairment can lead to either an inability to make decisions, or to the making of ill thought out decisions.

The Gall Bladder is paired with the Liver.

The Stomach

The Stomach Receives and Stores Food

The Stomach has the function of receiving food, separating out the pure essence that it passes on to the Spleen where it is refined into Gu Qi and passing on the impure to the Small Intestine for eventual excretion.

The Stomach Qi Descends

The natural function of the Stomach is to send Qi downwards for further processing. If this function is in any way impaired, then the Stomach Qi is said to be 'rebelling upwards'. This leads to belching, hiccups, regurgitation, nausea and vomiting.

The Stomach is paired with the Spleen.

The Small Intestine

The Small Intestine Separates the Pure from the Impure

The Small Intestine receives partially digested food from the Stomach. The pure is extracted under the control of the Spleen and the impure is then passed either to the Large Intestine or to the Bladder for excretion. The Small Intestine also performs this function with the Body Fluids.

The Small Intestine is paired with the Heart.

The Large Intestine

The Large Intestine Absorbs the Pure and Excretes the Impure

The Large Intestine receives the impure from the Small Intestine, which it further refines to extract any further pure fluids or essence and excretes the impure as faeces.

The Large Intestine is paired with the Lungs.

The Bladder

The Bladder Stores Urine and Controls Excretion

The Bladder receives waste body fluids from the Lungs, the Small and Large Intestines and under the influence of the Kidneys it stores and excretes this as urine.

The Bladder is paired with the Kidneys.

The San Jiao

The San Jiao Coordinates Transformation and Transportation of Fluids in the Body

The San Jiao coordinates water functions in the upper, middle and lower Jiao areas of the body. The San Jiao can perhaps be likened to the manager who oversees the workings of his or her 'team'.

The San Jiao Regulates the Warming Function of the Body

By ensuring that the Yang energy of the Kidneys is coordinated appropriately, the San Jiao helps move Qi and maintain the ambient temperature in the body. This function is recognized in its alternative names the Triple Heater, Triple Burner or Triple Warmer.

The San Jiao is related to the Pericardium.

THE FUNCTIONS OF THE EXTRA FU

As if the Zangfu were not enough to be contending with, Chinese medicine also talks about the Extra or Extraordinary Fu (sometimes referred to as the Curious Fu).

They resemble the Fu in as much as they are considered hollow, yet they have functions of storage that relate them more to the Zang. They tend to store the Yin essences of the body, namely, Jing, Marrow and Blood.

We can very briefly mention their functions:

- The Uterus regulates menstruation and promotes conception. (There is considered a male equivalent in the Dan Tien area called the Jing or Semen Palace.)
- The Brain stores Marrow – it is known as the 'Sea of Marrow'.
- The Marrow nourishes the bones and fills up the Brain.
- The Bones store bone marrow.
- The Blood vessels contain the Blood.
- The Gall Bladder is also considered an Extra Fu since it has a storage function with Bile.

This brief mention of the Extra Fu is included here merely for completeness – they will not be discussed in any further detail.

THE ZANGFU – CONCLUSION

We have been on a brief, but thorough, tour through the main structural underpinnings of Chinese medicine. The reader wishing to find out more should consult the Bibliography.

Armed with this understanding of the Zangfu, we can now look at how this is used to understand what is happening when our bodies start to give us problems.

5

The Causes of Disharmony

H AVING SET OUT a description of the elaborate system that Chinese medicine uses to understand the body and its processes, it will be clear that the concept of this system existing in a dynamic equilibrium is absolutely central. So little is said about structure and so much about process that the idea of imbalance does not seem unusual.

The more mechanistic view of Western medicine leads us continually into a way of thinking that equates illness with something that has caused some aspect of our biological mechanism to 'break down'. This inevitably leads on to treatment approaches that focus primarily on the damaged 'bit'. Now there are occasions where this view is appropriate and where it leads to valuable and effective treatments, but it does create a psychological set that can be counter-productive at times.

Chinese medicine, on the other hand, begins to think of disease as arising from influences that have disturbed the harmony and the balance of the whole energy system and although they may appear as symptom specific, we are encouraged never to lose sight of the 'balanced whole'. In this chapter we will look at the influences that Chinese medicine considers important when disharmonies occur.

For the purposes of our discussion, the causes of disharmony will be divided into three broad areas:

- Internal Causes
- External Causes
- Miscellaneous Causes

THE INTERNAL CAUSES OF DISHARMONY

As will have been clear from Chapter 4 on the Zangfu system, Chinese medicine considers the internal organs as influencing not only the physical functions of the body but also the psychological and spiritual aspects as well. The major internal causes of disharmony are considered psychological in nature and are termed the seven emotions. These seven emotions are:

- anger
- joy
- sadness
- grief
- pensiveness
- fear
- fright

In some instances there are clear overlaps between some of these emotions and with certain pairs the distinction is more a matter of degree, for example sadness and grief; fear and fright. As always, Chinese medicine does not neatly compartmentalize emotions and such overlaps are not considered problematical.

Relating back to the Five Element correspondences, the emotions can be associated with the organ system as follows:

Emotion	Zang	Fu
Anger	Liver	Gall Bladder
Joy	Heart	Small Intestine
Sadness ⎫ Grief ⎭	Lungs	Large Intestine
Pensiveness	Spleen	Stomach
Fear ⎫ Fright ⎭	Kidney	Bladder

Thus, in effect, when considering the relationship to the five Zang and their related Fu, the seven emotions are considered to be five.

Clearly, the experience of emotion is intrinsic to the human experience, and in Chinese medicine these emotions are as important in maintaining health as they are in creating potential ill health. It is always seen as a matter of degree. If there is an excess or a lack of emotional expression in any area, then this is what is likely to lead to disharmony. The seven emotions are considered neither 'good' nor 'bad'; it is how they balance out in an individual's life that is considered important. Thus, for example, too much joy is considered just as imbalanced as too much grief, it is simply that the disharmony will present in a different way.

We can now briefly consider each of the seven emotions in turn and consider how they may lead to disharmony.

Anger

Anger in this sense covers the full range of associated descriptions including resentment, irritability and frustration, among others. Anger will affect the Liver, resulting in the stagnation of Liver Qi. This can lead to the Liver energy rising to the head resulting in headaches, dizziness and other symptoms. In the long run it can result in high blood pressure and cause problems with the Stomach and the Spleen.

Joy

In Chinese medicine the concept of joy more readily refers to a state of agitation or over-excitement, rather than the more passive notion of deep contentment. The organ most directly affected here is the Heart. Such over-stimulation can lead to problems of Heart fire leading to such symptoms as feelings of agitation, insomnia and palpitations.

Sadness and Grief

The Lungs are most directly involved with these emotions. A normal and healthy expression of sadness or grief can be expressed as a sobbing that originates in the depths of the Lungs – deep breaths and the expulsion of air with the sob. However, sadness that remains unresolved and becomes chronic can create a disharmony in the Lungs, making the Lung Qi weak. This in turn can interfere with the Lungs' function of circulating the Qi.

Pensiveness

In Chinese medicine, pensiveness is considered to be the result of over-thinking or too much mental and intellectual stimulation. Any activity that involves a lot of mental effort will run the risk of causing a disharmony. The organ most directly at risk here is the Spleen. This can lead to a deficiency of Spleen Qi, in turn causing worry and resulting in fatigue, lethargy and inability to concentrate. This can be exacerbated by the fact that individuals with such a pattern often have poor and irregular eating habits that can also damage the Spleen.

Fear and Fright

Fear is a normal and adaptive human emotion, but when fear becomes chronic and when the perceived cause of the fear cannot be directly addressed then this is likely to lead to disharmony. The organ most at risk here is the Kidneys. In cases of extreme fright the Kidneys' ability to hold Qi may be impaired leading to enuresis. This can be a particular problem with children. Kidney Qi may become depleted leading to a deficiency of Kidney Yin. This in turn will lead to symptoms of empty heat including night sweats and a dry mouth.

Most people experience a wide range of emotions that vary in intensity. Some are appropriate and adaptive, others less so. It is important to be aware of how these emotions may influence the balance of Qi in the body and how this may exacerbate disharmonies.

THE EXTERNAL CAUSES OF DISHARMONY

In Chinese medicine there are considered to be six external causes of disharmony that relate to climatic conditions. They are variously known as the six pernicious influences, the six pathogenic factors or the six outside evils. They are:

- Wind
- Cold
- Damp
- Fire and Heat
- Dryness
- Summer Heat

In temperate climates such as those in northern Europe, the most commonly observed factors are Cold, Damp, Wind and to some extent Heat. However, we will discuss each in turn.

Wind

Wind is considered a Yang pathogenic influence. Wind is considered to have similar characteristics in the body as it has in nature. Most especially:

- Wind causes movement.
- Wind causes sudden change.
- Wind causes shaking and swaying.

Wind is a very influential external factor and has the effect of penetrating the exterior of the body and can often combine with other external factors – especially Cold – to invade the body. Wind disharmonies are often characterized by their sudden onset. A very common condition related to Wind is the common cold. If the Wei Qi is weak then Wind and Cold can readily penetrate the surface of the body and rapidly penetrate to the most 'external' of the internal Zang, namely the Lungs. This leads to the classic symptoms of sneezing, shivering, free flowing clear mucus and so on. It is interesting to note that if the Wind–Cold disharmony takes hold then the cold symptoms will turn to heat symptoms – as Yin transforms into Yang. Thus, the disharmony will change to fever, sore throat, dry mouth and yellow, thick phlegm and so on.

In Chinese medicine, Wind can also be related to an internal disharmony, usually to do with the Liver. Internal Liver Wind tends to be a much more serious disharmony and can result in conditions such as epilepsy, stroke or Parkinson's disease. The internal Liver Wind rises and causes the body to shake and tremble.

Wind is related to the Spring according to five element correspondences and this suggests that in Chinese medicine an individual is more likely to be susceptible to external Wind disharmonies in the Spring.

Cold

Cold is considered a Yin pathogenic influence. Its main effects are:

- Cold constrains movement.
- Cold constrains warmth in the body.
- Cold causes contraction of the body.
- Cold can lead to stagnation.

An invasion by Cold will be of sudden onset and will leave the individual feeling chilly, headachy and with an aversion to cold. The body may generally ache and there is likely to be no evidence of sweating.

If not dealt with, invading Cold can affect the Lungs as stated before, but also the Stomach and the Spleen, possibly leading to abdominal pain, vomiting or diarrhoea. It can also affect the Liver channel, especially in the genital area causing pain and discomfort.

Internal Cold usually results from a chronic Yang deficiency that may have a variety of causes, one of which would be long-term exposure to external Cold.

As might be expected, Cold is associated with the season of Winter.

Damp

Damp is considered a Yin pathogenic influence. The idea of Damp in Chinese medicine shares many of the qualities that would be associated with damp in the environment, notably:

- Damp is wet.
- Damp is heavy and lingering.
- Damp is slow to clear.

When damp invades the body it leads to sluggishness, tired and heavy limbs, muzzy headedness and general lethargy. Any body discharges will tend to be sticky and turbid and the tongue will tend to have a sticky coat. The Spleen is especially susceptible to Damp, which will inhibit the transporting and transformational functions of the Spleen. This can lead to abdominal distension and possibly diarrhoea. Damp can affect the joints, leading to stiffness – especially in the morning on rising, and they can become aching and swollen as is found in some arthritic conditions. Damp also tends to readily combine with both Cold and Heat.

If the Spleen becomes damaged due to invasion by external Damp or possibly through poor diet, this can lead to a more chronic internal Damp condition that can lead to the accumulation of Phlegm. Internal 'invisible' Phlegm can be particularly problematical in Chinese medicine, contributing to such problems as chronic dizziness and hypertension (high blood pressure).

In the Chinese calendar, Damp is associated with the late Summer, which can be wet. However, it is reasonable to see that Damp can occur at any season of the year depending upon the local climatic conditions.

Fire and Heat

In Chinese medicine it is not unusual to use the terms Fire and Heat interchangeably. They are considered Yang pathogenic influences. The characteristics of these influences are fairly obvious:

- Fire and Heat are hot.
- Fire and Heat induce movement.
- Fire and Heat are drying.

Fire and Heat lead to a whole plethora of heat type symptoms, including fevers, inflammation, red eyes, aversion to heat, hot skin eruptions and so on. They have a very drying effect on the Body Fluids with dry skin, constipation, yellow and scanty urine as common examples. Fire and Heat can also lead to disturbing psychological patterns, including hyperactivity, mental agitation and, in severe cases, delirium and mania. This is due to the Heat disturbing the Shen.

There can also be internal Fire and Heat conditions. A Yin deficiency, usually termed 'Empty Heat', will affect a number of Zangfu organs, although in all instances there is usually an underlying Kidney Yin deficiency.

Fire conditions tend to be associated with the Liver, the Stomach and the Lungs and lead to conditions where Fire blazes upwards, often affecting the head. For example, Stomach Fire can result in acute toothache as the Fire rises up the Stomach channel to the face.

Fire and Heat are associated with the Summer, heat stroke being a good example. Obviously, there will be climatic variations that will influence this. However, individuals who live in cool, damp climates are potentially quite susceptible to invasion by Fire and Heat if they go to a hot country, on holiday say, and do not take appropriate precautions.

Dryness and Summer Heat

We will consider these last two external influences together. They are much less common and less important than the others discussed above. Both are considered Yang pathogenic influences.

Dryness is really on a continuum with Heat and the symptoms are similar, but with a greater emphasis on the drying up of Body Fluids. It can lead to cracked skin, dry lips and nose and a dry cough with little or no phlegm. The Lungs can be particularly susceptible especially if the heat is accompained by a drying wind.

Dryness is associated with Autumn, but again this is geographically specific.

Summer Heat is associated with the height of Summer and again is on a continuum with Fire and Heat. It is often associated with very hot and humid climates, thus adding an element of Damp. It readily depletes the Qi and Body Fluids leading to exhaustion and dehydration.

As can be seen, the external cause of disharmony represents the environmental experiences that go along with living. Which factors individuals will be exposed to will depend on the climate where they live, but nevertheless the extent to which the factors will lead to disharmonies will be a function of the general robustness of an individual's Qi and their behavioural patterns. None of us can avoid exposure to these influences, but how we look after ourselves will to a large extent determine how they affect us.

MISCELLANEOUS CAUSES OF DISHARMONY

In addition to the main internal and external factors that have been described, there are a number of other factors that need to be taken into consideration. These will be briefly outlined below.

Constitutional Factors

As was discussed under a consideration of Basic Substances (Chapter 2), Chinese medicine recognizes that an individual's energy system comprises Pre-Heaven Qi and Jing as well as that produced through life. Our pre-heaven inheritance represents our constitution, which is a function of our parents. If the pre-heaven inheritance is deficient then this will leave the individual more susceptible to the whole range of external and internal factors, which can cause a disharmony.

If we believe that we have any constitutional weakness then particular care needs to be taken to ensure that other potential causes of disharmony are avoided or at least minimized.

Lifestyle Factors

We are all aware of the general stresses that accompany normal daily life and Western medicine readily recognizes that these 'life factors' can be very influential in terms of health and well-being. Chinese medicine similarly recognizes the importance of lifestyle, although this will be interpreted in a different manner.

Work

The kind of work we do – or the lack of work in the case of someone who is unemployed – can have a profound influence on our energy system. Too much physical work can impair the Qi and with excessive lifting the Lungs become deficient. Too much mental activity can damage the Spleen and make the Yin deficient. Someone who works out of doors is more liable to be at risk from Cold, Damp, Wind or Heat and so on.

Exercise

The amount and kind of exercise we take can have an influence, not to mention the lack of exercise that can cause Qi stagnation over time. As with everything in Chinese philosophy, it is a matter of balance. It is not a matter of any particular exercise being good or bad, but if the exercise is undertaken to an extreme this can cause a clear disharmony. For example, many athletes who train to an excessive degree and on the face of it appear very fit, are often very susceptible to infections and injuries. In the long run they may become chronically Qi deficient due to over-stressing the Kidneys. It will be noted that many of the Chinese exercise regimes such as Qigong and Taiqi are not obviously aerobic in nature like many Western forms of exercise. They do, however, offer a more balanced approach to exercise consistent with the principles of Chinese medicine. Good health and longevity are a notable feature of the practitioners of such activities.

Diet

Diet is afforded a very important place in Chinese medicine and a discussion of diet is a whole book in itself (see Bibliography). The Stomach and the Spleen have the responsibility for processing the ingested food and extracting the Gu Qi, which is then passed to the Lungs as a central part of the production of Qi in the body. If the Spleen has to work against poor and damaging foods then it will suffer – especially from damp – and the knock-on effect will deplete the Qi of the whole body. Again, balance rather than specific do's and don'ts represents the Chinese approach to diet. If an individual follows a healthy balanced diet, then the Spleen will remain healthy and the Qi of the body will be sufficient. The over-emphasis on sweet and processed foods in many Western diets does not lend itself to such a balance.

Sexual Activity

In Chinese medicine, excessive sexual activity is considered to be damaging to the Kidney Jing leading to long-term deficiency problems. Excessive childbirth can seriously deplete the woman's Blood and Jing.

There are various prescriptions as to what is excessive sexual activity, but generally the Chinese system emphasizes this naturally reducing as part of the ageing process.

Unforeseen Events

The last general category that should be mentioned includes accidents and injuries, which obviously can affect the Qi of the body depending on their type and severity. The Chinese would also consider events such as plagues and epidemics as belonging here and although they may be a problem in certain parts of the world, they are generally not an issue for the West. But we have plenty of other problems such as pollution and contamination of food which can readily be placed in this category.

CONCLUSION

Whether they are internal emotions, external pernicious influences – avoidable and unavoidable – what is clear is that the experience of living offers many ways in which disharmonies in the body can occur. Chinese medicine recognizes the manner in which a whole cocktail of influences can conspire together to create patterns of disharmony in the individual.

A Self-reflective Exercise

This chapter has highlighted the ways in which Chinese medicine sees disharmonies occurring in the body; some internal causes, some external causes, some avoidable, some less so.

In this exercise you are invited to consider yourself, your lifestyle and your environment and make a judgement about the areas of 'risk' from the perspective of Chinese medicine.

Internal Factors

For each of the seven emotions give yourself a score on a five-point scale as follows:

1. I handle this emotion very well.
2. I handle this emotion quite well most of the time.
3. Sometimes I handle this emotion well, sometimes I don't handle it well at all.

4. I do not tend to handle this emotion too well.
5. I handle this emotion very badly.

Emotion	Score
Joy	
Anger	
Grief	
Sadness	
Pensiveness	
Fear	
Fright	

You might find it interesting to have a friend or relative – someone who knows you well – complete this about you as well. The comparison of opinions can reveal a lot!

Look at the final pattern that emerges. It will give you a very rough guide to where disharmonies may occur and what Zangfu may be affected as a result of your internal factors.

External Factors

Consider the environment you live in. Consider the climate, any pollution that may be endemic, and then complete the following five-point scale:

1. I never experience this external factor.
2. I rarely experience this external factor.
3. I experience this external factor sometimes.
4. I quite often experience this external factor.
5. I very often experience this external factor.

External Factor	Score
Wind	
Cold	
Damp	
Fire/Heat	
Dryness	
Summer Heat	
Pollution (specify)	

This will give an idea of the potential external factors that you are susceptible to and by considering the information in this chapter you will get some idea of the kinds of problems that may arise if you do not look after yourself.

Reflect on your responses to this very simple questionnaire. Do not take it too seriously. As with any of these kinds of exercise, all it can do is offer some very general pointers that you may wish to be aware of.

Disharmonies in the body are neither necessary nor inevitable. The Daoist tradition was to seek longevity with health and well-being. To live a full and active life and to die healthy requires awareness and action, not luck!

6

Diagnosis and Patterns

THE PRACTITIONER OF Chinese medicine is confronted with the problem of trying to make sense of the myriad of processes that are going on within the individual. The need to have a systematic way of organizing all the information is of great importance if treatment plans and strategies are to be implemented successfully.

Some general approaches to diagnosis will be discussed and several of the more commonly used frameworks for organizing such information will be considered.

DIAGNOSTIC APPROACHES

The need to gather valid and comprehensive data is a *sine qua non* of any assessment process regardless of whether the problem is a burst pipe, a job applicant, a broken-down car or an unwell person. Without this assessment information it is impossible to formulate a hypothesis of what is going wrong and what to do about it.

In Chinese medicine the diagnostic process is considered in four areas – the four examinations. These four areas are:

- Looking
- Hearing and Smelling
- Questioning
- Touching

Each of these four areas will reveal information that when brought together will build towards a comprehensive whole.

Looking

The first thing that the practitioner of Chinese medicine will seek to do is to observe the patient and note anything about his or her physical appearance that may be of significance. To a large extent, this is something that we all do all the time with each other and we make intuitive judgements about a person's health based on observed data. For example, 'You look well today', 'Are you a bit under the weather?' and so on. We observe general demeanour, face colour, the condition of someone's hair, without really thinking about it. Chinese medicine seeks to do this in a more systematic way.

These are some of the more important aspects of looking.

Physical Body Appearance

A strong healthy-looking body is likely to have a strong internal organ system and is less likely to suffer from a deficient condition than a weak and frail body. Very thin people may be prone to Blood and Yin deficiencies, whereas obese individuals tend towards Qi deficiency and internal dampness.

The way a person moves can provide useful information. Fast and jerky movements suggest an excess condition or heat, whereas slow, deliberate movement suggests deficiency or cold.

The condition of the hair can give information about the Lung condition and premature balding and greying indicate deficiencies of Blood and of Kidney Jing.

The colour and the general appearance of the face are important. Some of the more significant aspects are:

- pale and lined face suggests chronic deficiency problems;
- puffy white face suggests Qi or possible Yang deficiency;
- red face indicates some evidence of internal or external heat;
- bags under the eyes suggest a Kidney disharmony;
- purple or blue lips can indicate a stagnation of Blood and may be related to a serious disharmony.

The condition of the skin can be important:

- dry skin suggests Blood deficiency;
- itchy skin suggests internal Liver wind;
- if the skin is swollen (oedema) this can indicate Qi stagnation or a deficiency of Kidney Yang

Tongue

Observation of the tongue is a central plank of Chinese medicine. It is not possible here to describe this most important aspect of 'Looking' in great detail, but there are some general points that can be made.

The 'geography' of the tongue is considered important. Various areas relate to the condition of specific internal organs as shown in Figure 18.

By observing the tongue condition in each of the areas, information is gathered regarding the condition of the relevant organ.

The important tongue characteristics are given in the following table:

Characteristic	*Significance*
pale red tongue	normal
pale tongue	deficient condition
red tongue	presence of internal heat
purple tongue	stagnation of Blood
blue/black tongue	internal cold present
thin tongue	deficient condition
swollen tongue	internal damp present
stiff or deviated tongue	internal wind present
quivering tongue	Spleen Qi deficiency
short horizontal cracks	Spleen Qi deficiency
toothmarks at side	Spleen Qi deficiency
shallow midline crack (not to tip)	Stomach deficiency
long deep midline crack (to tip)	Heart condition present
thin white coating	normal
thick coat	presence of pathogenic influence
no coat/tongue peeled	Yin deficiency present
white coat	Cold present (normal when thin)
yellow coat	Heat present
slightly moist	normal
wet tongue	internal damp present
sticky coat	phlegm present
dry tongue	Heat present

Figure 17. Tongue characteristics

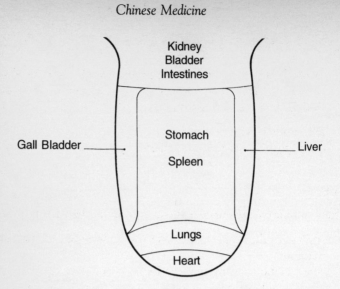

Figure 18. The 'geography' of the tongue

Hearing and Smelling

Listening to the patient's voice can be useful. A loud, penetrating voice tends to suggest an excess condition, whereas a quiet voice is more indicative of a deficient condition. Talking too much may be a sign of heat, whereas an unwillingness to talk suggests the presence of cold.

In a similar manner, the sound of the person's breathing can suggest an excess or a deficient condition.

The extent to which practitioners engage actively in smelling their patients is likely to be limited – especially in Western cultures, but some general points can be made. The presence of a strong unpleasant smell tends to suggest the presence of heat, whereas no smell at all usually suggests cold. If the urine and faeces are foul smelling this suggests presence of heat and possibly damp as well.

Questioning

A lot of information is gathered by asking the patient a series of questions and considering the answers with respect to the principles of Chinese medicine. There are various aspects that are usually covered in the course of a diagnostic interview.

Ears

The ears relate to the Kidneys in Chinese medicine and problems with hearing may indicate a Kidney disharmony. Tinnitus can be evidence of a Kidney or Liver disharmony:

- high pitch suggests Liver disharmony;
- low pitch suggests Kidney disharmony.

Eyes

There are various features of the eyes that can be useful:

- pain can indicate Heart or Liver disharmony or an external Wind invasion;
- 'floaters' and blurring suggests Blood deficiency;
- pressure and/or dryness could suggest Kidney disharmony.

Nose, Throat and Chest

These areas of the body relate to the Lungs and the Heart most directly.

- chest pain may suggest stagnant Blood or Wind-Heat invasion if there is associated cough and yellow, offensive phlegm;
- chronic blockage and stuffiness suggest damp and phlegm.

Trunk and Abdomen

The location on the body of pain or discomfort can suggest specific organ involvement:

- hypochondrium/flank relate to Liver and Gall Bladder;
- Epigastrium relates to the Stomach and the Spleen;
- Lower abdomen can indicate Liver, Bladder or Kidney disharmonies.

Head

In Chinese medicine the head is the confluence of all the Yang channels. If there is an excess of Yang energy coming to the head this can lead to problems such as headaches and dizziness. If there is a deficiency of Yang then this can lead to lightheadedness or possible unconsciousness. A detailed differential description relating to channels and Zangfu involvement goes beyond the scope of this book, but suffice it to say that detailed information regarding disharmonies in the head area is very important in Chinese medicine.

Digestion

This area of questioning can help focus on the Spleen and the Stomach.

- lack of appetite suggests Spleen deficiency, whereas constant hunger suggests Stomach heat;
- taste in the mouth can point to a variety of possible disharmonies, usually of the Spleen and Stomach, but also of the Kidneys and the Liver.

Drink and Fluids

An area clearly related to diet is the individual's thirst. The important thing to consider is the type and amount of fluids taken in. Generally:

- drinking cold liquids suggests a Heat pattern and vice versa with warm liquids;
- no thirst suggests a Spleen disharmony with Cold;
- thirst but lacking a desire to drink suggests Damp-Heat;
- sipping slowly usually suggests Yin deficiency.

Bowels

The nature of bowel movements is an important indicator of possible disharmonies in the body:

- constipation may suggest Heat, Cold, Blood deficiency or a Liver-related disharmony;
- diarrhoea may suggest Heat, Spleen, Kidney or Liver disharmonies.

Acquiring detailed and accurate information about bowel movements is very important in Chinese medicine.

Bladder

Features of passing urine are also of considerable importance:

- difficult urination suggests a Kidney or Bladder disharmony;
- frequent urination suggests deficiency of Kidney Qi;
- pain on urination suggests stagnation or heat; pain after urination suggests a deficiency problem;
- colour of urine suggests Cold if clear, Heat if dark and Damp if cloudy;
- extremes in the amount of urine passed suggests a Kidney disharmony.

Sleep and Energy Patterns

The pattern of the patient's sleep and energy are pointers towards the health of the Qi, Blood and the Yin of the body. The nature of insomnia suggests a varying pattern of disharmonies:

- not getting to sleep easily relates to Blood deficiency;
- continually waking and sleeping indicates a Kidney disharmony;
- dream-disturbed sleep suggests either a Liver or Heart disharmony;
- waking very early suggests a Gall Bladder disharmony;
- falling asleep during the day or general lethargy and low energy suggest a Spleen disharmony or possibly a Kidney disharmony if the problem is very severe.

Sweat

The characteristics of any pattern of sweating can be very helpful in discriminating disharmonies. There are various important factors:

Area of body affected, for example:
- head only suggests Stomach heat;
- soles/palms/chest ('Five Palm Sweat') suggest Yin deficiency.

Time of day, for example:
- day-time sweat suggests Yang deficiency;
- night sweats suggest Yin deficiency.

Pain

It is always important to ascertain the location, duration and nature of any pain that the patient may be suffering. Again, a description of the full differential diagnostic features of pain goes beyond our discussions here, but some important aspects are as follows:

Pain due to an excess condition is usually acute, sharp and specific. It may be due to:

– invasion by external influences;
– interior Cold or Heat;
– stagnation of Qi, Blood or Phlegm due to external injury or a Zangfu disharmony.

Pain due to a deficient condition is usually dull, achy, more chronic and more generalized. It may be due to:

– Qi or Blood deficiency.

The location of pain will give pointers to the affected channels that can be of importance both for exterior and interior disharmonies.

Response to Climatic and External Factors

This area of questioning really relates to the effect that external Heat, Cold, Damp or Wind has on the individual. This can lead to an understanding of any internal disharmonies that may be present:

– dislike of Cold and like of Heat suggest a Cold pattern or perhaps a Yang deficiency (particularly common in older people);
– dislike of Heat and like of Cold suggest a Heat pattern or perhaps a Yin deficiency;
– dislike of Damp suggests a tendency to Dampness;
– dislike of Wind may suggest a Liver disharmony, particularly as it relates to Liver Wind.

Emotional Features

It is always important to try and ascertain any disharmonies that may be associated with the individual's emotional state. As was pointed out earlier, the seven emotions are central to the concept of how disharmonies occur in Chinese medicine and an understanding of how the patient responds emotionally can give indications concerning any potential area of disharmony and the Zangfu system that may be involved. In particular consider:

– evidence of anxiety; may suggest Heart pattern and disturbed Shen;
– evidence of depression; may suggest Lung or Heart disharmony;
– evidence of anger/frustration; may suggest a Liver disharmony;
– evidence of poor concentration; may suggest a Spleen disharmony;
– evidence of undue fear; may suggest a Kidney disharmony.

Lifestyle Features

It is very important to be clear about aspects of the patient's life that may contribute to any pattern of disharmony. In particular, information should be gathered about:

- diet;
- exercise patterns;
- smoking, alcohol consumption;
- family and relationships;
- occupation and hobbies;
- drugs and medication taken (legal or illegal).

Such information may help build up the picture that explains the nature of the disharmonies that the patient presents with. For example, tension in a relationship can lead to anger and frustration that in turn may cause the Liver Qi to stagnate. In a situation such as this, a treatment programme may include a referral to Relate for marriage counselling in addition to Chinese medical treatment. There would be little point in using acupuncture, say, to move the stagnant Liver Qi if the underlying cause is not addressed, that is, the relationship difficulties.

Gynaecological Features

In gaining an accurate diagnostic picture with women it is important to explore the gynaecological patterns. Again, this is a detailed area in itself and beyond the scope of this book, but the following general points would be explored:

- regularity of menstrual cycle;
- amount of blood loss during period;
- colour and consistency of menstrual blood;
- menstrual pain;
- related premenstrual symptoms (if any);
- leucorrhoea.

Touching

The last aspect of the Four Examinations involves the practitioner working 'hands-on' with the patient. There are two aspects of touching that need to be considered: palpation of the body and taking the pulse. Pulse-taking is considered such an important aspect of Chinese medicine that a whole mystique has built up around it raising it to the level of an art form rather than an aspect of diagnosis.

We will consider both aspects of touching, but look at palpation first.

Palpation

Palpation refers to the systematic feeling of the surface of the body in order to discover any external or internal disharmonies. There are three main aspects of palpation.

Body Temperature

It can be useful to correlate the patient's report of whether he or she feels hot or cold by feeling the skin, generally:

- if skin feels cold then this suggests a Cold disharmony;
- if the skin is hot to the touch then this may suggest an invasion by external Heat;
- if the skin begins to feel hot after holding for a while then this may indicate internal Heat, possibly due to Yin deficiency.

Body Moisture

Again, it can be useful to correlate the patient's report of sweating and moisture by direct feeling of the skin:

- moist skin may suggest a Lung disharmony;
- dry skin may suggest a deficiency of Blood or Body Fluids.

Pain

An important indicator of areas of stagnation can be gained by palpating along the meridians looking for possible tender spots – 'Ashi' points as they are called in Chinese medicine. They may indicate a local channel problem or may be indicative of a more deep-seated Zangfu disharmony. It should also be borne in mind that many acupuncture points are naturally tender when they are palpated strongly and as such may not indicate any disharmony. Any such palpation information can only be considered in conjunction with all other aspects of a diagnostic picture.

Pulse

As stated above, taking the pulse is considered to be of prime importance in Chinese medicine. The emphasis is on the quality of the pulse in various positions on the wrist. There are recognized to be some twenty-eight different pulse qualities that can be felt on three different positions and at three different depths on the wrist of each hand – each with its own subtle nuance of interpretation.

Clearly, a full understanding of pulses in Chinese medicine is beyond the scope of this book, or any other, for that matter. Any fledgling practitioner of Chinese medicine soon learns that understanding pulses is more of an art, requiring practical experience. It would be similar to trying to learn to swim from a book – impossible!

With that important preamble in mind, we will explore some of the basic aspects of the pulse in Chinese medicine.

Pulse Position

There are three positions near each wrist on the radial artery. Each position relates to a specific aspect of the Zang organs. This is shown in Figure 19.

Pulse Depth

The depth at which the pulse is felt is also considered important. There are three levels, which each require slightly increased pressure. This can be illustrated in Figure 20.

Pulse Rate

As in Western medicine, the speed of the pulse is taken and compared with the average range of about 68–75 beats per minute.

Position	Left wrist	Right wrist	Energy
First	Heart	Lung	Qi
Second	Liver	Spleen	Blood
Third	Kidney Yin	Kidney Yang	Yin

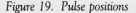

Figure 19. Pulse positions

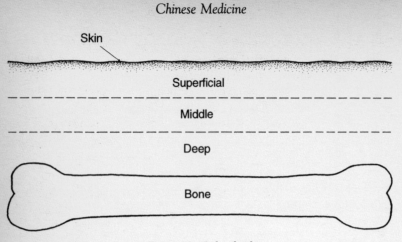

Figure 20. Pulse depth

Pulse Width

The width of the pulse between the fingers is noted.

Pulse Strength

An important indicator of whether a disharmony is an excess or a deficiency can be gained from judging the strength of the pulse.

Pulse Quality

There are a variety of qualities to the 'feel' of the pulse that are considered indicators of a particular disharmony pattern.

Pulse Rhythm

The consistency of the pulse flow and the nature of any inconsistency are considered important.

In the table opposite, the major features of the most common pulses are given. Again, it should be remembered that this is offered as an exemplar of a topic that is considerably more complex.

There are other less common pulse qualities that could be described, but the table gives a breakdown of those most commonly observed.

Diagnosis and Patterns

Pulse	Characteristic	Significance
floating or superficial	more apparent at surface, lacking at middle and deep level	invasion by external factor – Cold; Wind and so on
deep	more apparent at deep level; lacking at surface and superficial level	internal disharmony
rapid	fast pulse, significantly above average	internal Heat
slow	slow pulse, significantly below average	internal Cold
thready/ thin	feels like a very fine thread under the fingers. Quite distinct	Blood deficiency
large/big	feels very broad but distinct under the fingers	excess condition
empty	feels similar to a large pulse, but lacks the distinctiveness	Blood and Qi deficiency
full	feels similar to a large pulse, very powerful at all levels	excess condition
wiry	feels taught and distinct beneath fingers; like guitar string	Liver disharmony
slippery	'slips' along under the fingers; like a viscous fluid	internal Damp; Spleen disharmony
choppy	feels uneven; like fingers bobbing on surface of sea	Blood deficiency
tight	similar to wiry pulse, but feels like a vibrating cord	excess condition; stagnation
irregular/ knotted	slow; may skip a beat on an intermittent basis	Heart Blood disharmony
intermittent	skips beat regularly	Heart disharmony (serious)

Figure 21. Pulse characteristics

It should also be noted that an individual's pulse can exhibit several qualities in different positions and depths and a full diagnosis may involve having to consider the qualities observed in relation to the appropriate organ defined by the position.

There are stories of Chinese master physicians who can diagnose the whole pattern of an individual's disharmony from feeling the pulses and nothing else. These stories may be apocryphal or there may indeed be a few unique master practitioners with this level of skill. For the majority of practitioners of Chinese medicine the development of the art of pulse diagnosis is a slow and painstaking process requiring years of practical experience. The pulse ultimately is taken as one, albeit very important, piece in the overall jigsaw that makes up the Chinese medical diagnosis.

CONCLUSION

As can be seen, a diagnostic process in Chinese medicine is an extremely comprehensive and complex set of procedures. The four examinations allow the practitioner to build a very full picture of the energetic and physical landscape of the patient and to develop subsequently a comprehensive treatment plan.

Invariably, in any diagnostic 'story' there will be some contradictory indicators that may appear to stand in opposition to what other findings suggest. The balance of probability is likely to win out and decisions will usually be made based on the 'best fit' set of diagnostic indicators.

PATTERNS OF DISHARMONY

Having gathered what is a very comprehensive set of information during the diagnostic process, the practitioner of Chinese medicine requires a way of organizing it so that it will make the overall understanding of the energetics and disharmonies as clear as possible.

There are several organizational patterns which can be used in Chinese medicine. These include:

- Eight Principle Patterns
- Zangfu Patterns
- Five Element Patterns
- Channel Patterns
- Six Stage Patterns
- Four Level Patterns

It is not the intention to discuss all of these patterns here. The most commonly used patterns are the Eight Principles applied to the Zangfu system, Five Element Patterns and Channel Patterns, especially with relatively simple external conditions.

In this chapter we will look at the Eight Principle Patterns and we will see how this can be applied to the Zangfu system (see p. 91) to describe more accurately the nature of internal disharmonies.

A number of acupuncturists will use the Five Element system to organize their diagnosis, but this system will not be described in this book. The Eight Principles approach as applied to the Zangfu system tends to be the dominant model used in China and increasingly in the West. Any reader interested in the Five Element approach should refer to the Bibliography.

The Eight Principle Patterns

The Eight Principles consist of four mutually interdependent pairs of characteristics. These are:

- Yin and Yang
- Interior and Exterior
- Cold and Hot
- Deficiency and Excess

This approach of using bipolar qualities is very much in keeping with the general Daoist philosophy of Yin and Yang, as described earlier in the book.

To be strictly accurate, this system considers Yin and Yang to be superordinate qualities which subsume the other three pairs, thus:

Yin	*Yang*
Interior	Exterior
Cold	Hot
Deficiency	Excess

We can consider the general characteristics that would be associated with each of the eight principles in Figure 22 over the page.

Combinations of Patterns

It should be remembered at all times that the Eight Principle Patterns are not considered to be discrete categorizations, they are simply a systematic way to organize a lot of information about a very dynamic energy system – the human body. If disharmonies appeared in neat

Principle	Characteristic Symptoms
Exterior	sudden onset; acute disorder; invasion by external pathogenic influences – Heat, Cold, Damp and so on; channel problems; floating pulse; head and neck symptoms rather than whole body
Interior	all other types of condition; whole body symptoms; chronic problems; *Zangfu* system affected
Cold	pale; aversion to cold; slow, deliberate movement; heat helps problem; introverted; clear urine; tendency to diarrhoea; pale tongue; whitish coat; slow pulse
Heat	reddish complexion; fever; rapid movement and speech; dislike of heat; cold helps problem; thirst; dark urine; tendency to constipation; reddish tongue; yellow coat; fast pulse
Deficiency	tiredness and lethargy; weak, insipid movement; weak breathing; quiet voice; pressure can relieve discomfort; poor appetite; pale tongue; empty pulse
Excess	heavy movement; loud voice and breathing; pressure exacerbates discomfort; thick tongue coat; large pulse
Yin	considered an amalgam of Interior, Cold and Deficiency characteristics
Yang	considered an amalgam of Exterior, Heat and Excess characteristics

Figure 22. The Eight Principle Patterns

compartments like the eight principles then practitioners of Chinese medicine would have a relatively simple job in analysing a patient's problem. The reality is, of course, that there always appear combinations of patterns that can shift and change like a kaleidoscope.

For example, a patient may present with evidence of invasion by Wind–Cold, which is an Exterior/Excess pattern, with Cold predominating. If not treated, the Wind–Cold will turn to Wind–Heat (the Yin aspect turning to Yang), which is an Exterior/Excess pattern, with Heat predominant. It is possible that the Exterior condition could become internal, probably affecting the Lungs. Over time the Lungs may be weakened resulting in a Qi deficiency. Thus, the problem will become an Internal/Deficient pattern, with once more the Yin aspect becoming dominant over the Yang.

There are certain combinations of patterns that are quite commonly seen, but these are fluid and changeable over time. It is vital that the practitioner of Chinese medicine uses the Eight Principle Patterns in a flexible way to keep track of the changing matrix of energetic balances and imbalances.

The more commonly observed pattern combinations are given below. In each case the pattern of symptoms will reflect the features of the combination, subsumed under the overall perspective of whether the pattern is predominately Yin or Yang. It is not intended to give detailed descriptions of each of the combined patterns here. Some will emerge in the case studies presented later in the book. The interested reader may wish to try and work out what they think these combined patterns will be like.

Exterior Cold (Excess)

This is a combination of a Yang and a Yin pattern and as a result these will mediate each other. The resultant combined symptoms will not be too extreme.

> Tony wakes up feeling slightly shivery with his body aching. His nose is running with a clear, thin discharge. He decides that bed is the best place for him that day!
>
> In the above simple example, the pattern is also Excess in nature, but in some instances there may be an element of Wei Qi deficiency and a more Exterior/Deficient pattern may occur. This is more likely to be a situation where the symptoms are perhaps more chronic but less severe. If Tony, for example, had a tendency towards deficiency then he may feel as if these symptoms were continually coming and going and occasionally flaring up. This might be the kind of individual who may be described as generally 'under the weather' and susceptible to all minor ailments. Thus, even in a combined pattern that is fairly clear, there may be other patterns that are contributing to the overall picture.

Exterior Heat (Excess)

This is a combination of two Yang patterns and the result will be a strong Yang pattern. The symptoms are likely to be much more extreme with Yang features predominant.

Despite staying in bed for the day, Tony begins to develop a rasping sore throat and he has an elevated temperature. He is sweating, bringing up thick, yellow phlegm. His pulse is rapid. He feels lousy and remains in bed.

As with the first example, the likelihood of the Wind–Cold developing into Wind–Heat may also be a function of the individual's underlying deficiency pattern.

The following patterns relate to Internal conditions.

Excess Cold

This is a combination of a Yin and Yang pattern that will mediate the overall pattern. If pain is present, the Excess pattern will result in this being intense and very sensitive to the touch.

Derek has been raiding his mother's freezer and he ate a whole tub of ice cream. He is complaining of severe cramping pain in his abdomen and has been to the toilet with acute diarrhoea. His mother's sympathies are stretched to the limit!

It is likely that the intense Cold of the ice cream has invaded the Stomach and Spleen setting up an Excess Cold pattern. Derek should recover fairly quickly and hopefully won't raid the freezer again in a hurry!

Deficient Cold

This is a combination of two Yin patterns and the resultant pattern will present as strongly Yin in nature. In clinical practice this is usually seen as a feature of chronic Yang Deficiency, usually affecting the Spleen or the Kidneys, creating a relative excess of Yin in the body. It can also occur in Heart and Lung patterns.

Margaret is 79 and lives alone on her pension. She finds it difficult to make ends meet in terms of food and heating at home. She is constantly complaining of being cold, even in mild weather and has little or no energy to do anything. She eats and drinks very little and suffers from chronic diarrhoea, especially first thing in the morning. Her ankles are swollen and her back is constantly cold and aching.

This is a classic example of the Kidney Yang energy becoming deficient as a feature of the ageing process and this is further exacerbated by Margaret's poor diet and lack of heating at home. In extreme cases in old age, the Yang energy becomes so deficient that coma and death follow – hypothermia.

Excess Heat

Both the patterns here are Yang in nature, so the resultant combination pattern will be markedly Yang in presentation. They will generally present with classic Heat signs and extremely dominant behaviours.

> Bill does not suffer fools gladly, and would get very frustrated and angry when things were not working out the way he planned. He was subject to episodes of extreme temper, where he would get very red in the face and invariably complain of thumping headaches. Bill was on medication for high blood pressure and his GP has warned him that if he doesn't slow down a bit he will end up having a stroke.
>
> Bill's anger and frustration were causing his Liver Qi to stagnate. This creates internal heat in the Liver that builds up and rises to the head as Liver Fire on occasions. Bill died of a massive CVA at the age of 51.

Deficient Heat

This is a combination of a Yin pattern and a Yang pattern and they will relatively mediate one another in the combined pattern. This pattern is most commonly seen as a result of a deficiency in Yin energy, resulting in a relative excess of Yang. This pattern is often referred to as 'Empty Heat' and is characterized by 'Five Palm Sweats', night sweats and a general mental agitation.

> Pauline has been going through the menopause and is having tremendous problems with hot flushes and night sweats. She complains of a constant nagging low back pain and she is continually feeling 'on edge', as if she is going to bite everyone's head off for no good reason. She is tearful and depressed at times and her sleep pattern is poor.
>
> A feature in menopause is the deficiency of Kidney Yin that results in the 'empty heat' symptoms that Pauline is experiencing. In addition, the empty heat is invading the Heart and disturbing the Shen causing the restlessness and the emotional symptoms.

The above represents the most commonly noted combined patterns. What should be noted, however, is that in any given individual it is perfectly possible for combinations of apparently opposite patterns to coexist. Thus, it is possible that an individual will present with a problem that is excess in nature, but that there also exists an underlying deficiency pattern. A general rule of thumb in treatment programmes would be to treat any excess patterns first and then move on to treat any deficient condition. These combinations will become clearer hopefully in the case studies that follow later in the book.

CONCLUSION

As has been seen, the taking of a diagnosis and the subsequent 'ordering' of the information in Chinese medicine is a complex and ever varying process. The emphasis is on change and how change influences the patterns of disharmony that are observed. When a treatment programme is planned and implemented it has to be applied with a constant eye on the complex, and at times contradictory, nature of change in the energy patterns of the body and how they influence the physical.

A Self-reflective Exercise

As a way of trying out some of these principles, you may wish to reflect on your own experience of illness – minor and perhaps not so minor – with respect to the Eight Principle Patterns. Do not take this exercise too seriously, you are not a trained practitioner and you will not be able to fully grasp the complexities behind our disharmony patterns.

However, take a piece of paper, and write down the headings as below:

- Exterior
- Interior
- Cold
- Hot
- Deficient
- Excess

Consider any signs and symptoms that you may recall and decide which principle categories they belong in. Once you have completed all this decide if any of the combinations seem to be possibly present. Finally, try and classify your disharmony as predominately Yin or Yang in nature.

You may, for example, decide that your problem is one of Interior Deficiency which is predominately Yin in nature.

If you feel that you do have a problem that you would like help with, then go to see your own doctor, or contact a fully qualified and registered practitioner of Chinese medicine. Information on how to obtain details of such practitioners is given at the end of the book.

Zangfu Patterns

The Principle Patterns outlined in the previous section provide a very helpful way to organize diagnostic information, but when the focus is on Interior Patterns it can be observed that disharmonies of Yin/Yang, Cold/Heat and Excess/Deficiency arise typically in certain consistent patterns affecting the Zangfu system. Thus, a further level of organizing patterns that can prove useful is to consider these consistent patterns as Zangfu 'syndromes'. The danger in solidifying a diagnosis into a syndrome is exactly that which results in the criticism of Western syndrome diagnostics. Once a syndrome becomes identified it carries the danger of becoming solidified into a 'thing' that the person has 'got' and this can lead to losing sight of the dynamic nature of energetic disharmonies. In order to avoid this danger, we will use the term Zangfu Patterns, which will help to keep a focus on the dynamics of change.

With this warning heeded, it can be shown that the Zangfu Patterns provide the practitioner with a further very useful level of subtlety and sophistication in making a diagnosis and then planning a subsequent treatment programme. There are far more Zangfu Patterns than can reasonably be dealt with here and consequently one of the most commonly occurring patterns from each of the Zangfu will be selected for detailed description. In each case we will look at the pattern from the following perspectives:

- What would be the major signs and symptoms that would characterize the pattern?
- How can the pattern be seen in terms of the Principle Patterns?
- What are the pathological processes in terms of Chinese medicine?
- What factors are likely to contribute to the disharmony?
- What would be the principle of treatment in Chinese medicine?

Where treatment is referred to it should be noted that approaches to treatment will be discussed in greater detail in Chapter 7.

Patterns of the Zang Organs

The Lungs

The observed Lung patterns are summarized in Figure 23 (Lung Qi Deficiency will be discussed in greater detail).

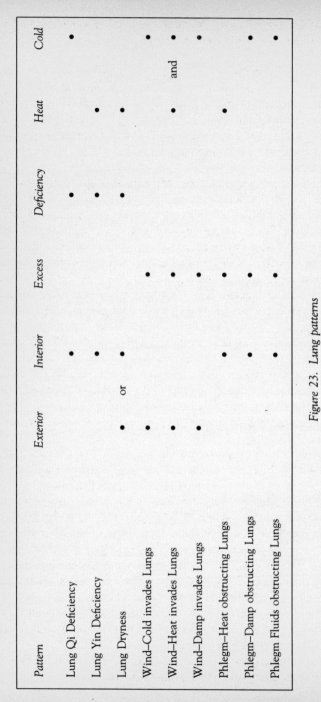

Pattern	Exterior	Interior	Excess	Deficiency	Heat	Cold
Lung Qi Deficiency		•		•		•
Lung Yin Deficiency		•		•	•	
Lung Dryness	• (or)	•		•	•	
Wind–Cold invades Lungs	•	•	•			•
Wind–Heat invades Lungs	•		•		•	• (and)
Wind–Damp invades Lungs	•		•			•
Phlegm–Heat obstructing Lungs		•	•		•	
Phlegm–Damp obstructing Lungs		•	•			•
Phlegm Fluids obstructing Lungs		•	•			•

Figure 23. Lung patterns

Lung Qi Deficiency   Problems of Lung Qi Deficiency are quite commonly observed, often exacerbated by pathogenic factors in the atmosphere.

Signs and Symptoms. There will be a shortness of breath, especially on exertion, and the voice will generally be weak and insipid. The complexion will be bright but pale white and there will be a tendency to sweat during the day. There will be a chronic cough with watery sputum. There will be evidence of general tiredness and lethargy and the individual will tend to be very susceptible to minor infections and ailments.

The tongue will tend towards pale and the pulse will be weak, especially in the Lung position.

Pathological Processes. When Qi is deficient, the Lungs fail in their function of governing respiration and as a result shortness of breath occurs in addition to weak voice. Qi will also not descend causing the cough, and the watery sputum results from the Lungs not regulating the water passages. When Lung Qi is deficient this will result in the Wei Qi being deficient also. This leads to sweating and a susceptibility to external pathogenic influences. The empty pulse indicates Qi deficiency.

Contributory Causative Factors.   There may be Pre-Heaven factors present here. Pre-Heaven Qi acts like a bank account which can be drawn from but not added to. Thus, if the parents' Qi is deficient, perhaps through disease such as TB or through habits such as heavy smoking, then their offspring are likely to have Deficient Pre-Heaven Qi, leading to a tendency to Qi deficiency which may weaken the Lungs.

People who work long hours in sedentary occupations that involve sitting crouched over a desk will restrict Qi flow in their Lungs due to bad posture and this can lead to Lung Qi deficiency.

The problem of Lung deficiency can be seriously exacerbated by invasion from Wind–Cold or Wind–Heat. If the body Qi is not strong enough to expel the pathogenic factors then this can injure the Lungs leading to Qi deficiency. Once the cycle becomes established, there is an increased risk of further invasions and, consequently, further Lung deficiency. Thus, a vicious circle can be set up that can lead to a chronic Qi deficiency problem. A point worth noting is that the tendency to give antibiotics for infections can lead to a serious impairment of the Lung's dispersing and descending function, further exacerbating the Qi deficiency.

Smoking will also damage the Lungs leading to Qi deficiency (and to Yin deficiency and other Lung disharmonies).

Treatment Principle in Chinese Medicine. It will be necessary to tonify the Lung Qi. In addition, the Yang energy can also be tonified.

This can be achieved using acupuncture, moxabustion or herbal preparation. In addition it would be important to avoid any habits such as smoking, and taking antibiotics would not be helpful, except in the case of very serious acute infections. The patient may also benefit from certain Qigong exercises, which will strengthen the Qi of the chest.

The Heart

The observed Heart patterns are outlined in Figure 24 (the Stagnation of Heart Blood will be discussed in greater detail).

Stagnation of Heart Blood   This condition in Chinese medicine is the parallel to a diagnosis of angina pectoris in Western medicine. The condition can be seen on its own and as a component of a 'Heart Attack'.

Signs and Symptoms. There will be palpitations and a stabbing pain in the chest area that may extend to the inner part of the left shoulder and arm. There may be a feeling of constriction in the chest. There may be shortness of breath and the symptoms are likely to be brought on or exacerbated with exertion. In severe cases there can be a blue/purple tinge to the lips and the nails. The hands will tend to be cold and possibly clammy.

The tongue will be very dark red or purple and there may be purple spots on the tongue body. The pulse is likely to be knotted.

Pathological Processes. This pattern is usually seen as a combined Excess and Deficiency pattern as the Blood stagnation will not arise on its own, but is likely to have resulted from Heart Yang or Heart Blood Deficiency. In some instances it can result from Heart Fire in which case it will be a uniquely Excess pattern. The actual pattern of symptoms will vary depending on what underlying pattern has been present.

When the Heart Yang energy is deficient this will result in insufficient Qi to move the Blood in the chest. The Blood will stagnate leading to the symptoms noted. As the Blood stagnates it does not reach the face and the hands, leading to the blue/purple colouring in the lips, tongue and nails. The deficient 'moving' energy in the chest causes the Heart beat to become irregular, exacerbated by internal Cold – palpitations and knotted pulse.

Contributory Causative Factors. It is generally seen that emotional

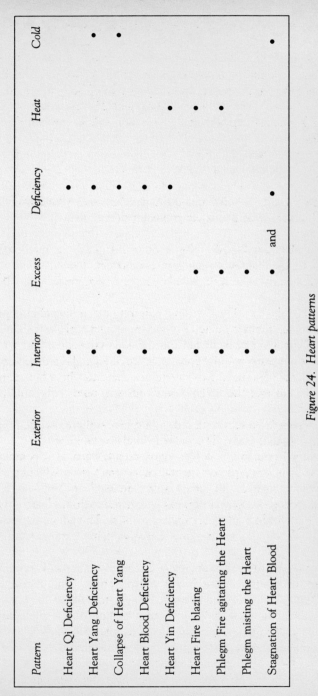

Figure 24. Heart patterns

factors play a strong role in creating Deficient Heart Qi, which can lead to Heart Blood and Heart Yang Deficiency over time. A poor diet may also exacerbate Heart Blood Deficiency. Anxiety is often 'stored' in the chest area and this can lead to Qi and Blood stagnation in that area.

Treatment Principle in Chinese Medicine. The treatment principle will vary depending upon whether the person is suffering a severe attack of stagnation pain, or whether the condition is less acute.

In the first instance the focus will be on moving the stagnant Blood and promoting circulation in the chest. In the less acute phase it is important to also tonify the Heart Yang and Blood and also calm the Shen.

In the acute phase acupuncture and herbal treatment may be used and this may be supplemented using moxabustion to tonify the Heart Yang in the more chronic phase.

Qigong exercises can be helpful in the chronic stage to tonify the Heart, and appropriate dietary advice should be followed.

The Spleen

The observed Spleen patterns are outlined in Figure 25 (Spleen Qi Deficiency is discussed in greater detail).

Spleen Qi Deficiency This disharmony is probably one of the most common that occurs in Chinese medicine. The pattern also underpins all other Spleen disharmonies and as such it is very important.

Signs and Symptoms. This condition is characterized by a general lassitude, poor appetite and a full sensation in the lower abdomen. There is likely to be a tendency towards diarrhoea and the limbs can feel heavy.

When the Spleen Qi becomes deficient this leads to a build up of internal Damp that can cause a feeling of fullness in the chest and epigastrium.

There can be a tendency for thought processes to become muddled with poor concentration. It is often described as trying to 'think through cotton wool'.

The tongue will tend to be pale or light pink and the sides of the tongue can be scalloped or toothmarked in chronic cases. There may also be transverse tongue cracks.

The pulse will be empty as characterizes a Qi Deficient condition. If there is a lot of Damp present, the pulse may be slightly slippery.

Pathological Processes. If the Spleen Qi is deficient this will impair the

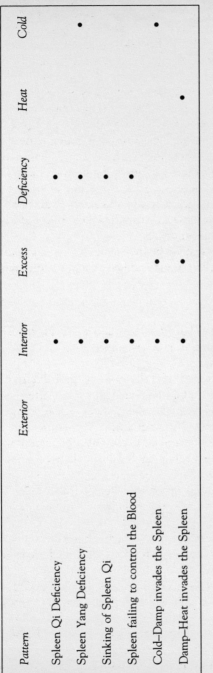

Pattern	Exterior	Interior	Excess	Deficiency	Heat	Cold
Spleen Qi Deficiency		•		•		
Spleen Yang Deficiency		•		•		•
Sinking of Spleen Qi		•		•		
Spleen failing to control the Blood		•		•		
Cold–Damp invades the Spleen		•	•			•
Damp–Heat invades the Spleen		•	•		•	

Figure 25. Spleen patterns

Spleen's ability to transform and transport food resulting in abdominal problems such as distension and loose stools. The Spleen will fail to send Gu Qi up to the Lungs and the overall Qi production of the body will be impaired leading to tiredness and lethargy.

The build up of internal Dampness causes stuffiness in the chest and epigastrium and can lead to feelings of nausea. As a result of the Spleen's link with thinking, a deficiency can lead to poor concentration and muddled thoughts.

Contributory Causative Factors. One of the main causes of this disharmony will be a poor diet. In particular an over-emphasis on cold and raw foods will impair the function of the Spleen and the consumption of low protein foods or a habitual 'dieting' pattern will further deplete the Qi.

Any mental strain will take its toll on the Spleen. Students who study a lot will cause the Spleen Qi to become deficient, as will mentally working while eating.

The other cause of Spleen Qi deficiency is over exposure to damp climatic conditions. Thus, people who work outdoors in a cold and damp climate, or in an artificially damp climate, will tend to become Spleen Qi Deficient.

Treatment Principles in Chinese Medicine. The focus of treatment will be tonifying the Spleen Qi. If there is evidence of Damp present, then treatment would also look at clearing Damp.

Acupuncture, herbal treatment and moxabustion can all be used to treat Spleen Qi Deficiency.

In order to strengthen the Spleen it is important to encourage a balanced, warming diet that avoids too much cold, raw and damp foods. Where there is lot of mental activity that could be contributing to the Qi deficiency, then a balanced approach encouraging exercise and resting should be recommended.

The Liver

The observed Liver patterns are outlined in Figure 26 (Stagnation of Liver Qi is discussed in greater detail).

Stagnation of Liver Qi Stagnant Liver Qi is one of the most common patterns seen by practitioners of Chinese medicine in the West – a large number of practitioners probably suffer the effects of this disharmony at some time or other as well!

Signs and Symptoms. There are a variety of physical and emotional characteristics associated with Stagnation of Liver Qi.

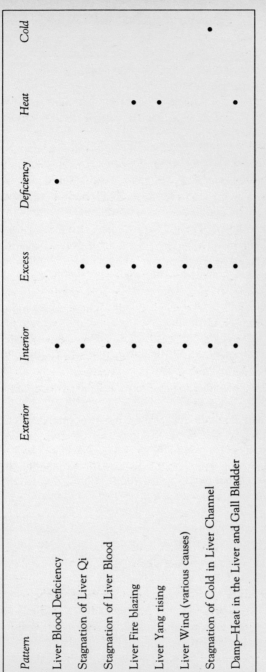

Pattern	Exterior	Interior	Excess	Deficiency	Heat	Cold
Liver Blood Deficiency		•		•		
Stagnation of Liver Qi		•	•			
Stagnation of Liver Blood		•	•			
Liver Fire blazing		•	•		•	
Liver Yang rising		•	•		•	
Liver Wind (various causes)		•	•			
Stagnation of Cold in Liver Channel		•	•			•
Damp–Heat in the Liver and Gall Bladder		•	•		•	

Figure 26. Liver patterns

There can be distension and discomfort in the flank area and, prior to a period, women may experience breast pain and distension. This discomfort may be accompanied by sighing and bouts of hiccuping.

There can be a tendency to epigastric upset, with nausea, vomiting, belching and some regurgitation of food. These symptoms may be accompanied by 'anxious stomach' sensation. There can be loose stools, but also at times the stagnation may result in constipation, especially with stools like 'round hard balls'.

There is usually a lot of emotional tension associated with stagnant Liver Qi and the individual may feel depressed, upset, tense and irritable. This can be accompanied by a discomfort in the throat, usually referred to as a 'plumbstone' throat.

Women may experience painful periods with dark red and clotted blood and premenstrual irritability.

The tongue tends to be a normal pink colour and the pulse is invariably wiry, especially on the Liver position.

Pathological Processes. The Liver Qi tends to stagnate in the flank area and the stagnation can be released by sighing. If the stagnation is more centred in the diaphragm area then hiccups tend to occur as they also move the stagnant Qi.

The emotional symptoms tend to reflect pent up anger and frustration, and this results from the fact that the Liver is not moving Qi and so anger, which is the emotion associated with the Liver, is not released. This also works in reverse in as much as if there is a lot of anger, frustration and resentment in a person's life, then this will have the effect of stagnating the Liver Qi. The depressive symptoms may initially suggest a Deficient condition, but this is not the case as the depression usually reflects the anger and resentment being turned in on the individual. An 'explosion' will eventually let it out. Stagnation of Liver Qi can appear like a malfunctioning pressure cooker – sooner or later the calm will be shattered in a very dramatic and violent manner!

The digestive problems result from the stagnant Liver energy invading the Spleen and the Stomach creating disharmonies in these Zangfu.

The 'plumbstone throat' and the tender breasts in premenstrual women result from the fact that the Liver channel flows through these areas and thus the stagnation is felt more acutely there.

The general menstrual problems arise because the stagnant Liver Qi impairs the Blood flow in the Chong and Ren channels, which govern the reproductive process in women.

In severe and chronic cases the Qi Stagnation can turn to Blood stagnation causing severe stabbing pain. This can typically occur in the Uterus and result in very painful periods for some women.

Contributory Causative Factors. The blame for Stagnation of Liver Qi is almost exclusively laid at the door of emotional factors. The strains and stresses of living can lead to frustrations in many walks of life and the social mores in Western cultures which emphasize holding back emotions and feelings can result in these emotions having nowhere to go. As a result this 'blocked emotional energy' clogs up the subtle energy system primarily affecting the Liver whose function it is to smooth the flow of Qi in the body. The result is Stagnation of Liver Qi.

Treatment Principles in Chinese Medicine. Treatment in Chinese medicine will focus on promoting the smooth flow of Liver Qi and dispersing the stagnant Qi.

Acupuncture can be very effective with this disharmony, as can herbal treatment. Exercise and Qigong practice can be very helpful in maintaining the natural flow of Qi round the body and thus coping with the stresses of everyday living that can so readily lead to Stagnation of Liver Qi.

The Kidneys

The observed Kidney patterns are outlined in Figure 27 (Kidney Yang Deficiency is discussed in greater detail).

Kidney Yang Deficiency Kidney Yang Deficiency is a common pattern, especially in older people when their Qi energy generally weakens.

Signs and Symptoms. This is a chronic Interior Cold disharmony and it is typically characterized by feelings of cold. It is especially notable in the low back area and in the knees.

The complexion is very pale, tending towards a bright white colour. There will be a poor appetite and chronic diarrhoea, which exacerbates the general feeling of tiredness and lassitude.

There can be infertility in women and impotence in men. There also tends to be copious quantities of clear urine and fluids gather under the skin causing oedema – especially in the legs and ankles.

The tongue will be pale and wet. Sometimes it will appear quite swollen. The pulse will be deep and quite empty or weak.

Pathological Processes. The deficient Kidney Yang energy will mean that the Mingmen Fire will fail to warm the body, resulting in the feelings of cold and also it will not nourish the Jing, resulting in the

Pattern	Exterior	Interior	Excess	Deficiency	Heat	Cold
Kidney Yin Deficiency		•		•	•	
Kidney Yang Deficiency		•		•		•
Kidney Qi not firm		•		•		
Kidney not holding Qi		•		•		
Kidney Jing Deficiency		•		•		
Kidney Yin Deficient with Empty Fire blazing		•	• and	•	•	
Kidney Yang Deficient with Water overflowing		•	• and	•		•

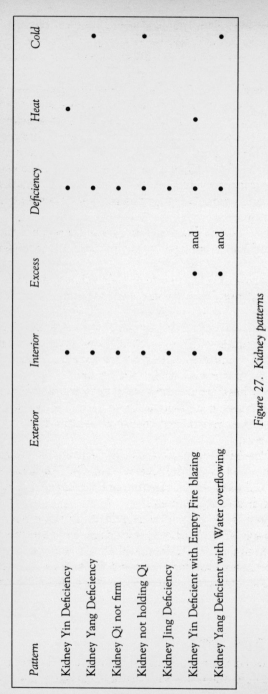

Figure 27. Kidney patterns

sexual disharmonies. The Kidneys have a role in strengthening and nourishing the bones and if the Kidney Qi is deficient, then there will be a tendency to aching, especially in the lower back around the Kidney area.

The Deficient Kidney Yang will fail to move the body fluids, resulting in the copious clear urination and also the accumulation of the Fluids under the skin leading to oedema. The diarrhoea is due to the Kidney Yang energy being insufficient to support the Spleen. The accumulated fluids will also show up on the tongue. In very severe cases the Yang energy may be so depleted that there is very little fluid movement and then the urination will be very slight. This is a good example of two apparently contradictory symptoms being consistent with the same disharmony.

Contributory Causative Factors. Kidney Yang deficiency may result from a chronic long-term illness that depletes the energies of the body.

Too much sexual activity can deplete the Kidney energy leading to Yang Deficiency, but this is a relative concept dependent on age and general health.

Kidney Yang Deficiency is a common feature of the ageing process and is quite common in older people. Old people quite often suffer from diarrhoea first thing in the morning, 'cock crow diarrhoea', resulting from very weak Yang energy when they get up.

If the Spleen has become chronically deficient over time, usually because of poor and inappropriate diet, then this can lead to the accumulation of internal Damp, which will ultimately damage the Kidney Yang energy.

Treatment Principle in Chinese Medicine. The main focus of treatment will be to warm and tonify the Kidney Yang Qi. This can be readily done using moxabustion or acupuncture with moxabustion, and certain Yang warming herbs may be useful.

It is also important to emphasize the role of diet and general lifestyle factors, such as avoiding drafts and cold, damp environments. Qigong exercises to strengthen the Kidneys will always be useful.

It should be noted that the Lungs and the Kidneys have a mutual support function, and to this extent it can also be helpful to tonify the Lungs as well.

Patterns of the Fu Organs

Although many common syndromes often relate to the five major Yin organs (the Zang), there are patterns of disharmony also associated with the Yang organs (the Fu). Space does not allow us to explore these in any detail, but the principles for identifying the disharmony, understanding the causative factors and planning an intervention, are the same as those for the Zang organs. The interested reader will find details of all Zangfu patterns in the Bibliography.

CONCLUSION

The above descriptions give a detailed insight into how the Principle Patterns can be further refined to look at patterns of disharmony relating to the Zangfu system in Chinese medicine. As can be seen, only exemplars have been drawn out to illustrate the kind of process that a practitioner of Chinese medicine will go through in looking at the range of signs and symptoms that the patient presents with.

In addition to the spectrum of Fu disharmonies, there are several other combined patterns that have not been mentioned. In such combined patterns there are characteristic linkages between the disharmonies of certain organs. For example, Kidney and Lung Yin Deficiency often occur together with a mutual reinforcement, one of the other.

It is also worth bearing in mind that any given patient going to a practitioner of Chinese medicine is going to present with several disharmony patterns at the same time. It becomes important that the practitioner be able to identify the various patterns that are occurring, whether they are Excess or Deficient, and plan a treatment programme accordingly.

The whole issue of planning and monitoring treatment programmes will be discussed in Chapter 7.

We can now begin to see how the unique insights and principles of Chinese medicine build up to form a logical and coherent body of knowledge that allows for help to be given in an equally logical and coherent manner.

We will discuss in Chapter 7 the forms of help that are available in greater detail.

What Patterns Can You See?

It may be useful and interesting to end this chapter by giving you, the reader, the opportunity to try and identify what patterns may be present in a given case history. Remember, this book is not offering anything that remotely approaches a training guide to Chinese medicine, but hopefully it can begin to help you 'think' in the way that a Chinese medical practitioner thinks.

Read the following case history carefully (it is a very straightforward one) and try to decide what you think is going on. Make a note of any signs or symptoms that you can identify and allocate them to the categories of the Eight Principle Patterns, namely:

- Interior
- Exterior
- Deficiency
- Excess
- Cold
- Heat

Decide if you think the condition is predominately Yin or Yang in nature. Finally, do you think the pattern that you identify can be associated with any Zangfu pattern?

> Maria is a 32-year-old physiotherapist. She is going through a very difficult divorce and is fighting over the custody of her two children with her estranged husband. In addition to this, she has recently been promoted at work and she is under a lot of pressure there to fulfil the expectations of her new job.
>
> She is complaining of feelings of abdominal distension, fullness in her chest and a constriction in her throat. She says that she has absolutely no energy and her legs feel like lead. She finds it difficult to lift and work with her patients. Her symptoms get worse prior to her period and she gets very moody and irritable with her children and work colleagues at this time.
>
> She says that her diet is 'OK', but she admits to being a bit obsessive about her weight and she eats a lot of salads at times and then binges on 'junk food', especially when she is very tense. As she puts it, 'whenever I have to talk to my husband, my diet goes right out the window!'
>
> Her tongue is a normal pinkish colour with slight toothmarks on the side. Her pulse is wiry.

Well, what do you think might be going on with Maria? Compare your ideas with the suggestions that I make in the Appendix (p. 140).

7

Treatment Approaches

H AVING SET OUT the underlying principles behind the Chinese
view of the human body and its dysfunctions, it is important
and appropriate to discuss the approaches that have been developed
to treat disharmonies of the energy body and facilitate the individual's
return to balance and good health. There are, however, some points
that should be made before saying any more about treatment.

The main point is that this is not a book on 'how to do' Chinese
medicine. The emphasis has been on trying to demystify the process
for the interested Western reader, not on offering simple do it yourself
tips. If nothing else has emerged from the previous chapters, then at
least it should be clear that Chinese medicine, while being logical,
elegant, subtle and holistic, is certainly not simple. It would be wholly
misleading to suggest that reading this book in any way prepares anyone
to actively treat a disharmony.

Therefore, when we discuss acupuncture, herbal remedies, moxabustion, cupping, acupressure massage, Qigong, diet and lifestyle in
the following sections, it will be informative to the extent that the
connection will be made between the treatments in general and the
underlying principles of Chinese medicine. However, acupuncture
point locations and prescriptions will be avoided, there will be
no information on what herbs to use in specific disharmonies, no
descriptions of specific Qigong exercises will be given and so on. All
uses of treatment protocols in Chinese medicine require appropriate
professional training and can be gleaned in only a very superficial way
from any book – no matter how thorough or well written.

Details will be given at the end of the book regarding where any
interested reader may get advice and information about professional
services in the area of Chinese medicine. Here, as suggested, we

will discuss acupuncture, moxabustion, cupping, herbal remedies, acupressure massage, Qigong, diet and general lifestyle factors.

PRINCIPLES OF TREATMENT IN CHINESE MEDICINE

Regardless of which treatment approach is decided upon, there will always be common aims and objectives. These aims and objectives form the principles of treatment and derive from the Eight Principle Patterns described in Chapter 6 and elaborated upon when Zangfu disharmonies were discussed.

A useful way to understand this may be to consider a simple analogy (see Figure 28). When a pressure cooker is operating efficiently, the pressure inside will be maintained at an optimum level in order to cook the food. This is achieved by ensuring initially the system is at an appropriate temperature and then using a simple valve to maintain the optimum pressure. The whole system is in dynamic equilibrium and the energy is used to achieve the ends for which the system was designed. However, problems can arise.

A Problem of Excess

Consider the situation if the valve blocks and the pressure inside the cooker rises beyond optimum. The system becomes unstable and unless some action is taken, there will be nasty consequences – the cooker will

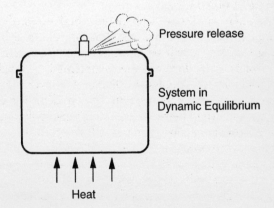

Pressure release

System in
Dynamic Equilibrium

Heat

Figure 28. Chinese medicine treatment as a pressure cooker

explode! It could be said that the cooker had experienced a condition of Excess and the reduction of this Excess is necessary in order to re-establish equilibrium.

A Problem of Deficiency

In this instance imagine that the valve is faulty and pressure is leaking away from the cooker at a faster rate than it is building. When this happens, it will take forever to cook the food or it may never cook at all if the pressure is lost altogether. What is required here is some way to tonify the system to once again build the pressure up to the optimum level necessary for equilibrium.

The analogy is simple to follow and it does not fully reflect the complexity of body energy processes, but it does give a very useful flavour to the essential aspects of what treatment is all about in Chinese medicine.

If there is a condition of Excess apparent in the disharmony, then it is necessary for the treatment to focus on *reducing* the Excess and getting rid of the factors – whatever they might be – that are causing the Excess in the first place.

If there is a condition of Deficiency apparent in the disharmony, then it is necessary for the treatment to focus on *tonifying* the Deficiency and ensuring that the energy is maintained at the appropriate level to ensure health and well-being.

The analogy can also demonstrate the Principles of Heat and Cold. The cooker requires a certain amount of Heat to work properly – too much or too little causes problems. Similarly, the body requires an optimum level of Heat to function efficiently. Too much Heat will lead to an Excess and too little will lead to a Deficiency. If too much Cold is present, this will also produce an Excess in much the same way that if the cooker were exposed to extreme Cold, its fluids (water) would freeze up, expand and cause severe damage.

Thus, if there is too much Heat in the body this should be expelled and if there is too little the body must be warmed.

The third way in which this analogy may help is in terms of the amount of fluid present. In the pressure cooker, if there is too much water added the food is liable to go mushy and lose its body. If it continues to be heated, the mush will dry out into an indigestible mess.

This would be analogous to there being too much Damp in the body. In time it can turn to Phlegm under the action of internal Heat. Just as the excess water should be drained from the pressure cooker, so the Damp requires to be drained (or resolved is the term used in Chinese medicine).

On the contrary, if there is too little water in the pressure cooker, the food will dry up and burn under the effect of being heated. It will become hard and possibly crumbly.

This would be analogous to the Body Fluids being insufficient and the effect is for the body to literally dry out and flake, for example, dry skin conditions. In this situation it would be necessary to promote the production of fluids and bring Heat to equilibrium level.

Now, these pressure cooker analogies should not be taken too literally, but they do give a sense of what treatment you might try to achieve in Chinese medicine. In summary:

- When a Deficiency exists, the energy should be tonified.
- When an Excess exists, the energy should be reduced.
- When too much Heat is present this should be expelled or cooled.
- When too much Cold is present this should be expelled or warmed.
- When Damp is present, this should be resolved.
- When Phlegm is present, this should be resolved.

As was pointed out before, patients often present with a mixture and complexity of disharmonies. In such instances the practitioner has to make decisions as to what aspects are the 'root' and what are the 'stem' – in other words, which aspects of the disharmony are more fundamental and which are more superficial. The treatment programme will then have to reflect the order in which these problems are to be dealt with. A common rule of thumb would suggest that Excess conditions should be treated before Deficiency conditions, but on occasions there may be exceptions to such a rule.

Ultimately, the aim of treatment in Chinese medicine is to ensure that the Yin and Yang energies of the body maintain their dynamic state of active equilibrium, thus promoting health and well-being in the individual.

TREATMENT APPROACHES

Acupuncture

The image of the body being pierced by fine needles in an apparent random way is perhaps the stereotypical view of Chinese medicine that is most commonly held by people. At face value, it must be difficult to relate this kind of treatment to the presenting condition for the vast majority. For the bulk of people, Chinese medicine will start and end with this image – forever arcane, bizarre and something to be doubted or feared.

The story may have ended there but for the fact that the Chinese have been using and refining the techniques of acupuncture for over 3000 years with consistent and remarkable effect.

It should be remembered that acupuncture has evolved as an empirical science – in other words, a knowledge base developed by the on-going and systematic observation of the effect of needling specific points and areas. Initially, crude needles made from animal bone and sharpened bamboo were used. It was noted that when they were inserted into 'ashi' points – points where pain was being experienced – then very often relief from the pain was obtained. Over subsequent centuries the energetic model of Qi, Jing, Blood and Fluids was articulated and the flows mapped as the meridians of the body. Specific points were identified and the actions of needling these points were recorded. The theory of acupuncture continues to develop and to be refined to this day.

As was suggested earlier, acupuncture points appear to offer access to the Qi flow of the body and when these points are stimulated by the insertion of fine stainless steel needles certain energetic and physical changes occur in the body.

The acupuncturist selects appropriate points for their specific actions in relationship to the identified disharmony. The point prescription is then needled and the needles may or may not be subsequently manipulated to achieve certain effects. The needles are usually retained in the body for between fifteen and twenty minutes, although this can vary from very short periods (seconds), often with children or infants, up to an hour or longer with certain stubborn patterns.

The needles can be manipulated by the practitioner to achieve the effect of tonifying the Qi – rotation or lifting and thrusting are the most common methods. On the other hand, other manipulations can be used to reduce the Qi in Excess conditions – often by slow insertion and quicker lifting. Other more 'even' techniques are neutral in their stimulation effect, which can be appropriate in certain conditions.

In certain Excess conditions, the needle reducing function can be stimulated by passing a minute direct current electrical pulse through paired needles.

Treatment protocols, frequency and duration are a matter of professional judgement for the practitioner, in consultation with the patient.

A common course of treatment may initially involve between ten and fifteen treatments spaced at approximately weekly intervals. The frequency could be less than weekly if the condition called for it, especially early on in a treatment programme, and may spread out to fortnightly or even monthly later in a programme.

Exacerbation of symptoms is a quite common feature of acupuncture treatment. In this regard, the patient may find that in the short term after treatment, the symptoms may in fact get worse before an improvement sets in. A professional practitioner will always warn the patient of the possibility of exacerbations at the start of a course of treatment.

Probably the majority of practitioners now use pre-packed and sterilized disposable needles that are used once, and only once, before being collected and destroyed by incineration. Some will still prefer to use re-usable needles that require to be sterilized to tight and rigorous standards after every time of use. All patients should enquire about types of needle used prior to treatment and if re-usable needles are being used they should ask to see the sterilization procedures that the practitioner adopts. In this time of HIV and related disorders, nobody – patient or practitioner – can afford to be anything other than scrupulous in terms of needle cleanliness.

Needles are available in varying lengths and varying 'thicknesses' or gauges. The choice of needle is usually determined by where the point to be needled is and what effect is being sought. Commonly used needles will vary in length from $1/2$ inch, through 1 inch, $1^1/2$ inch, 2 inch, up to 3 inch.

Needle sensations vary from dull aching pain to a tingling 'shock'. In some instances the sensation travels along the line of the meridian and can affect whole areas of the body or limbs. This can lead to feelings of heaviness in the limb. The patient may feel a bit tired or washed out shortly after a treatment, but this usually passes quite quickly. However, people vary in their reactions to acupuncture and some of these effects may be minimal or totally absent in some patients.

Acupuncture can be remarkably effective in many conditions that occur today. The effectiveness is strongly dependent upon a thorough and accurate Chinese medical diagnosis. The needling skills and techniques of the practitioner will also influence greatly the effectiveness of the outcome. The typical pattern in the West has seen the acupuncturist as often the last port of call for individuals with long-term chronic problems. Treatment, not surprisingly, was often slow and in some cases of marginal benefit. However, as acupuncture establishes itself more and more, it is becoming the treatment of choice for many people and the effectiveness of the approach with acute as well as with more chronic conditions is being increasingly recognized.

Moxabustion

Moxabustion is the process whereby a dried herb called moxa – usually the species mugwort (*Artemisia vulgaris*) – is burnt, either directly on the skin or indirectly above the skin over specific acupuncture points. The purpose of this process is to warm the Qi and Blood in the channels. Moxabustion is most commonly used when there is the requirement to expel Cold and Damp or to tonify the Qi and Blood.

As moxabustion puts heat into the body, it is clearly not indicated in conditions of internal Heat, and although it may be useful with exterior Excess conditions in the channels, generally it is not used for interior Excess conditions.

When lit, moxa burns slowly and provides a penetrating heat that can enter readily into the channels and influence the Qi and Blood flow. Moxa burns with a characteristic smell and can give off a fairly copious smoke. Some patients may find the smell and the smoke difficult to tolerate and the odour will be retained in clothing and hair long after a treatment session. Smokeless moxa is available, but this can be very difficult to light and is not commonly used.

Moxa is available in a loose form that can be used for making moxa cones. Alternatively, moxa is packed and rolled in a long stick like a large cigar, about 15–20 cm long and about 1–2 cm in diameter.

Direct Moxabustion

In this instance, the moxa is formed into small cones which are then placed on the selected point of the body and lit. The moxa cone is allowed to burn down almost to the skin, is then removed and a new cone added as necessary until the practitioner considers the treatment concluded. If it burns too far down, direct moxa can scar the skin and although practices exist where scarring is actively encouraged, this is not the practice in the West.

Indirect Moxabustion

More commonly, moxa is burnt indirectly, either above the skin or on another medium between the moxa and the skin.

Moxa cones can be burned on a slice of ginger, a slice of garlic or on a layer of salt. The choice of medium separating the moxa from the skin will depend on the condition being treated and the clinical opinion of the practitioner.

Moxa sticks can be lit and held above the area to be worked on. They will be turned in a rotational fashion or 'pecked' in and out, around the affected area for anywhere up to ten minutes. Care has to be taken not to touch the skin.

Moxa sticks can be cut into smaller pieces that can then be placed over the end of a stainless steel or copper-handled needle once it has been inserted into an appropriate acupuncture point. The moxa is then lit while on the end of the needle. In this way, the heat not only warms the skin but is also drawn into the channel through the needle. Loose moxa can also be wrapped onto the needle and used in the same way.

When heat is required over a more general area, for example, when there is low back pain due to stagnation of Qi in the channels, then lengths of moxa may be burnt on a metal grill within a moxa box, which is placed over the affected area.

Once again, the choice of when and where to use moxabustion, either on its own or in conjunction with acupuncture, is a matter of clinical judgement for the practitioner of Chinese medicine, but this should always be explained and shared with the patient beforehand.

Cupping

Cupping is a technique that is especially useful in treating channel problems resulting in localized stagnation of Qi, or in helping to expel the external pathogenic factors, Wind–Cold, which have invaded the Lungs.

Cups are either of robust rounded glass construction or of bamboo. Other materials have been used, but by far the most common type of cup used by practitioners in the West is glass. A typical glass cup is shown in Figure 29.

A vacuum is created inside the cup by burning a taper for a very short period of time in the cup and then immediately placing the cup down over the selected area. Because the taper flame exhausts all the oxygen in the cup a vacuum is created and this has the effect of 'drawing up' the skin beneath the cup. The effect of this is to encourage the flow of Qi and Blood in the area beneath the cup. By moving the Qi and Blood, local stagnation can be cleared. In the case of cupping to expel Wind–Cold, the cups would be placed over the lung area in the upper back. In appropriate cases, cupping can be carried out over an inserted acupuncture needle.

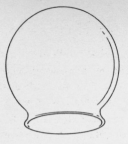

*Figure 29. A cup used to draw Qi and Blood to the surface of the skin
under a vacuum*

Cupping naturally draws blood to the external capillaries of the body
and as a result minor weals or bruises may be left after a treatment.
If the practitioner is using cupping then this should be explained as
a possible consequence of treatment.

Acupressure Massage

Massage is widely used in Chinese medicine and various different
techniques have been developed as part of the evolution of Chinese
medicine in general. In Chinese, massage is called *An Mo*, where *An*
translates as 'push' and *Mo* translates as 'rub'.

Acupressure can be used over general areas of the body to promote
the flow of Qi and Blood through the meridian system. This approach
can be invaluable for minor channel disharmonies involving a local
stagnation of Qi and Blood.

Cavity press massage concentrates on applying pressure to specific
acupuncture points in order to achieve specific systemic changes in the
body. In this instance, different forms of pressure are applied depending
on whether the aim is to tonify, to reduce or to achieve a more
neutral, calming effect. The choice of points used in any acupressure
prescription will be based on a differential diagnosis resulting from an
exploration of the patterns of disharmony as previously described.

Simple acupressure protocols can be given as a set of 'self-help'
techniques that individuals can use with themselves or with partners
and friends. Many minor ailments and disharmonies respond quite well
to simple acupressure and they can form the basis of simple Chinese
medicine 'first aid' (see Bibliography).

Acupressure massage techniques can be used in conjunction with
other approaches to treatment in Chinese medicine.

Chinese Herbal Medicine

Alongside acupuncture, herbal medicine is a major pillar of Chinese medicine. Herbal preparations have long been used in Chinese medicine and a comprehensive 'Materia Medica' can be found dating to about 650AD. As the knowledge base grew over the centuries more and more information regarding herbs and their properties was collected and in 1977 a modern compilation recorded some 5767 herbal entries in terms of their properties and the disharmonies that they were helpful with.

Herbs are classified in two major categories. The first category refers to the temperature characteristics of the herb, being one of:

- hot (re)
- cold (han)
- warm (wen)
- cool (liang)
- neutral (ping)

The second category refers to the taste property of the herb, being one of:

- acrid (xin)
- sweet (gan)
- bitter (ku)
- sour (suan)
- salty (xian)

The various combinations of temperature and taste give the herb its properties that can influence the Yin and Yang energy patterns of the body. Thus, there are herbs that will warm, herbs that will cool, herbs that will tonify, herbs that will move stagnation and so on.

Thus, when a Chinese herbal practitioner takes a diagnosis, there will be a description of disharmonies in terms of the affected Zangfu and the Eight Principle Patterns. Once the treatment principle has been decided upon, the practitioner will select appropriate herbs and combinations of herbs that will have the desired effects. Herbs can be prepared in the form of decoctions, powders, pills, syrups and plasters for external application.

The effects of herbal preparations can be very specific and it is important that the practitioner accurately diagnoses the disharmony and prepares the appropriate prescription in terms of the relative amounts and dose of specific herbs.

Patent herbal remedies in the form of pills, decoctions and teas are available for more general symptomatic treatments. These patent remedies are well tried and tested combinations of ingredients prepared in pill, capsule or decoction form. A growing number of preparations manufactured in the West are now supplementing traditional patent remedies from China.

As with Western drugs that can be bought over the counter without prescription, patent remedies can offer a more general effect that can be very helpful with less severe symptoms and disharmonies. However, their effects will, by their very nature, be less symptom-specific than the effect of a customized herbal prescription based on the pattern of an individual's disharmonies. Patent herbs are often used in combination with acupuncture treatment as an adjunctive therapy to support the overall treatment plan and facilitate a speedier recovery from the presenting disharmony.

Herbal remedies can be very effective with many disharmonies, but it is essential that any prescriptions are made by a fully qualified and registered practitioner in Chinese herbal medicine (see Useful Addresses).

Qigong Therapy

Probably one of the most dramatic growth areas in terms of Chinese medical practice in the West is the interest in Qigong. Bookstores are carrying a burgeoning range of titles on the subject, most of them offering simple self-help exercise regimes. There is nothing intrinsically wrong with this, but very little information is being offered regarding the linkage between Qigong exercises and the theory and practice of Chinese medicine. Many people are being attracted to Qigong through an interest in Taiqi, which despite the fact that its roots lie as a martial art, is essentially a form of moving Qigong and shares the same basic principles.

While this is not the place to discuss Qigong as a therapy in great detail, it is important to make some general observations in order to see it within the context of Chinese medicine. Without this background, Qigong is simply Chinese callisthenic exercise.

Qigong can be translated as 'energy cultivation' or 'energy development'. In terms of Chinese medicine, Qigong is the art of promoting the strength of the 'Three Treasures' – Jing, Qi and Shen through calming the mind, breath control, physical movements and stances. As will have been clear throughout the discussions in this book, the Chinese view believes that illness is a manifestation of a disharmony and weakness in the individual's energy system. Consequently, if the energy system is strong and balanced, there will be no illness. Thus, Qigong practices can be an invaluable aid in maintaining the vitality of the energy system and the health and well-being of the individual.

Qigong practices probably predate the earliest accounts of primitive acupuncture and may well have been used some 5000 years ago, or even earlier than that. Over this period of time, literally thousands of Qigong exercises and strategies were developed, handed down and refined through generations of families and practitioners. In the last twenty years or so, many of these practices have spread from China to the West and there is a growing articulation of Qigong as an important aspect of Chinese Medicine. Qigong practice is now being subjected to scientific research methodologies and there is a growing body of impressive evidence for the effectiveness of these practices.

There are two aspects of Qigong practice that can be considered and we will look briefly at both:

- Qigong exercises as a self-help preventative strategy.
- Qigong healing.

Qigong Exercises

Qigong exercises can be sub-divided into four main categories.

Static Exercises

In these exercises the individual will hold a variety of static postures, either standing, seated or occasionally lying down. Specific postures can relate to the strengthening of the energy flow in specific Zangfu systems or they can relate to the general energy flow of the body. These static exercises often appear deceptively simple, but they are inevitably quite demanding, some extremely so, and they usually require the practitioner to build up practice periods over an extended time scale.

Movement Exercises

These exercise forms can vary from relatively simple sets of movements, to the complexity and beauty of the various Taiqi forms or some of the more dynamic forms such as Dayan (Wild Goose) Qigong and Swimming Dragon Qigong, for example. Many of the movement forms (and static forms as well) are based on a translation into human movement of the natural and graceful movements of animals. Some of the postures within the Taiqi forms, for example, demonstrate this powerful imagery and connection – 'snake creeps down' and 'white crane spreads wings' being typical.

Breathing Exercises

Strong and appropriate respiration is essential for the promotion of healthy Qi flow in the body. The Chinese view is that we acquire external Qi from the air that we breathe and a variety of Qigong breathing exercises work to develop good breathing habits.

Meditation Exercises

Calming the Shen and ensuring that it remains housed in the Heart is essential in maintaining emotional harmony. Meditation practices teach the individual to focus on a calm and harmonious Qi flow throughout the body. In many respects, Qigong meditation practices differ little from many of the meditation approaches taught by other traditions.

In practice, several of the above aspects of Qigong practice are combined. Thus, for example, static exercises will also involve breathing techniques, as will meditation practice.

There are other practices within Qigong that introduce elements such as sound. For example, the 'Six Healing Sounds' is a form of Qigong that combines postures with the frequency and vibrational qualities of certain key sounds that are related to specific organ functioning.

Some of the simpler exercises and practices can be learned from a book, but for many – and ideally all – Qigong exercises, it is necessary to have guidance from an experienced practitioner. Unlike acupuncture and herbal medicine, where there are fully trained and registered practitioners, finding a Qigong teacher can be a real lottery. If Qigong is being taught at a simple level as a form of exercise, then it is likely that the movements will be little more than superficial bending, stretching and deep breathing. Now this will, of course, be of value in most instances, but it should not be presented as more than that.

However, anyone offering Qigong exercises to aid specific ailments should at least be a registered and experienced practitioner of Chinese medicine and ideally have some form of accredited Qigong training.

The latter is unlikely at this time, but as Qigong develops and is seen as a central plank of Chinese medicine, then this will become increasingly established.

Qigong Healing

Qigong healing is an altogether much more fascinating and controversial area of Chinese medical practice. In this, the practitioner emits his or her own Qi through key acupuncture points in his or her body to affect the Qi flow in that of the patient. This is done without any physical contact in most instances. There is a growing body of literature and evidence from China regarding the emission and the guidance of Qi by the Qigong practitioner and how this can be focused in the patient in order to facilitate Qi balance and to redress any presenting disharmony.

Central to this practice is the necessity for the practitioner to have a strong and robust energy system that will rely on the self-practice of many of the Qigong exercises and practices discussed above. There are also some quite specific hand gestures that are taught in order to emit Qi, for example; 'Five Thunder Fingers' and 'Spreading Claw' techniques.

In China, the practice of Qigong healing can be combined with acupuncture, where the Qi is guided to the specific acupuncture needles in order to enhance the therapeutic effect.

These practices are only now becoming better known in the West and for some individuals, even some practitioners of Chinese medicine, they represent a very challenging conceptual shift. It is likely that a lot more research and training will be required before such practices become a regular part of the treatment armoury of practitioners of Chinese medicine in the West.

As has been emphasized throughout this book, Chinese medicine operates at an energetic level that in turn results in changes at a physical level. No one reading this book should doubt that Qi emission and guidance is real. The corollary of this is that these are techniques that require a deep understanding of Chinese medicine, specific training and supervised experiential practice. If anyone offers Qigong healing then you must be very aware of the powerful energetic forces that are being worked with and consequently you should be quite clear about the qualifications and the experience of the practitioner.

The whole area of Qigong as a specific therapeutic approach in Chinese medicine is only now developing in the West and it has the potential to stand beside acupuncture and herbs as a major pillar of practice. In the meantime, many health benefits can be acquired by the regular practice of some simple Qigong exercises.

Diet and Lifestyle

As diet can be considered an aspect of general lifestyle, these two will be considered together. Chinese medicine is no different from Western medicine in recognizing the importance of lifestyle attitudes and behaviour patterns in the health and well-being of the individual. Therefore, any treatment strategy that is agreed between the practitioner and the patient will reasonably include advice regarding these factors.

Diet

The issue of diet in Chinese medicine can be considered on two levels:

• healthy dietary patterns
• dietary treatment regimes

We will discuss briefly each in turn.

Healthy Dietary Patterns

As with everything else in Chinese medicine, appropriate diet is a matter of balance. The Middle Jiao is the area of the body that deals with digestion, extracting the Gu Qi from the ingested food and sending it up to the Lungs. The general vigour of this Middle Jiao area is maintained through diet and the vitality of the food eaten is central to this process.

Food is considered to have both internal and external energetic qualities. In terms of the internal qualities, any given food can be energetically hot, warm, neutral, cool, cold and damp. In addition to this the food will have externally defined qualities of heat and cold depending upon whether and to what extent it has been cooked.

It is generally felt that the Spleen requires to be warm, but not too hot, in order to carry out its functions with respect to digestion. Thus, Chinese medicine would suggest that it is beneficial for food to be primarily cooked and to contain slightly more energetically warming foods, so as to promote the healthy function of the Spleen and the Middle Jiao. Limited fluids should be taken with a meal and the food should be adequately chewed to ensure efficient digestion. Over-eating will lead to an impairment of Middle Jiao function and should be assiduously avoided. Cold and raw foods, especially frozen ones, should be taken only sparingly. The other factor that would be relevant as far as food is concerned would be climate and season. In the cold damp weather of the winter it is important to ensure a diet of energetically warming foods. A general rule of thumb would see an ideal healthy diet as consisting of cooked warming foods, with the avoidance of extremes. The common practice in the West of seeing a diet of salads and raw foods as being beneficial would be seriously questioned within the Chinese system. One of the Chinese doctors under whom I trained used to berate patients who were vegetarians on the grounds that such a diet is imbalanced and will inevitably lead to Qi deficiency. Needless to say, this is a rather generalized position, but it does point to the manner in which Chinese medicine will take a somewhat different emphasis when it comes to diet.

Food represents potential Qi which the body has need of. Thus the quality of the food in addition to its energetic properties and how it is cooked is also important. Stale and processed foods should be avoided where at all possible as the Qi will be greatly diminished. Similarly, food that is left over and re-heated, especially if refrigerated or frozen, will be significantly lacking essential Qi. It need hardly be said, but the majority of mass prepared 'fast' and 'junk' foods so readily available in the West, score so abysmally on all counts that their essential Qi is virtually non-existent.

Ideally, food should be organically prepared, lack any additives and be as free as possible from pollutants or insecticides. Good Chinese cooking emphasizes the use of fresh produce at all times, where the cooking time is minimal in order to allow the food to retain the highest quality of essential Qi.

It is not necessary, nor is it desirable, for people in the West to try and follow a wholly Chinese approach to food preparation and diet. It is useful, however, to be aware of the needs of the body from an energetic point of view when it comes to food and to be aware, as far as possible, of the energetic qualities of the food being eaten.

Above all, follow a well-balanced, predominantly cooked diet and don't eat too much!

Specific advice regarding books on diet from a Chinese medical perspective are given in the Bibliography.

Dietary Treatment Regimes

When we come to consider dietary advice that is a specific part of a treatment protocol, it has to be remembered that we are operating right on the borderline between diet and herbal treatment.

As stated before, foods are considered to have energetic qualities in exactly the same way that herbs are. Thus, various foods or food combinations may be recommended by a practitioner of Chinese medicine with a view to addressing a specifically identified pattern of disharmony. Thus, for example, carrots may be recommended to Tonify the Spleen and to Resolve Damp and pork may be recommended to Tonify Qi, Blood and Yin.

Clearly, any practitioner recommending a pattern of foodstuffs and diet to address a specific disharmony should have appropriate training and background in Chinese medicine.

Lifestyle

In addition to diet, there are a whole range of lifestyle issues that will be pertinent, both in formulating a diagnosis from the perspective of Chinese medicine and also in planning a treatment strategy. Some of these factors will be within the control of the patient, some will not be. None will be within the control of the practitioner. Some of the more common lifestyle factors are discussed below.

Relationships

Relationships at home, at work or with people in general, can be of tremendous importance when considering energetic disharmonies. On the one hand, good relationships can be a vital support in overcoming an illness, whereas bad relationships can undermine even the most comprehensive and well-planned treatment strategy.

Difficult relationships can cause anger and frustration and can thus lead to the stagnation of Liver Qi, with all that potentially can flow from that. General unhappiness and anxiety can disturb the Shen, leading to problems such as insomnia.

The practitioner may point out the contribution that relationship difficulties may be having towards the patient's disharmony and a referral to another professional such as a counsellor or psychologist may be suggested.

Addictions

Various substances can fall into this category, but the most common ones that will be seen by practitioners of Chinese medicine are smoking and alcohol. Although they are clearly different in many respects and their long-term abuse will result in different disharmonies, there are some energetic similarities. Both are energetically Hot substances and they will put heat into the body. In the long run this can be very damaging, but in the short run there can be some energetic benefit that leads to the addiction. The main feature here is that the heat will tend to move stagnant Qi and where there is Liver Qi Stagnation with all its associated symptomatology, the taking of tobacco or alcohol will temporarily move the stagnant Qi, so producing a short-term beneficial effect. Once the effect has worn off, the Qi stagnation returns and so a vicious circle is set up.

The practitioner may have to decide in any given situation whether tackling the addiction is an immediate priority or whether it is something that can be returned to at a later stage. Either way, it may well be important to support the patient in dealing with such addictions as part of a treatment programme. Chinese medicine can help directly, for example acupuncture can be very helpful in aiding smokers giving up, or it may involve referral onto other professionals or voluntary groups.

More serious addictions such as drug abuse will in themselves almost certainly be a central feature of the patient's disharmony pattern and require to be treated as such.

However, it should be remembered that in all examples of addiction the practitioner of Chinese medicine does not have magic solutions and the attitude and willingness of the patient to address the problem is vital in gauging potential treatment effectiveness.

Exercise

Physical exercise, or the lack of it, can be very important in working with some disharmonies. Generally speaking, moderate physical activity is a very good way to move Qi and Blood and so to promote a smooth energy flow around the body. The corollary of this can be that a lack of moderate physical activity can lead to a sluggishness in the body and can create stagnation and possible Qi deficiency. There will be many instances where a practitioner will wish to recommend moderate physical activity such as swimming, walking and cycling, for example. There is much less of a tendency to promote very vigorous activity, as this may lead to the creation of disharmonies. For example, too much running can lead to the body becoming Qi deficient, potentially leaving the individual susceptible to other problems.

Physical Environment

A brief mention of this may be appropriate here, especially given the growing interest in the Chinese practice of Feng Shui. This is not the place to discuss this in any detail but suffice it to say that the logic of the Chinese system suggests that the energy flow associated with where we live, the way we orientate and decorate our rooms, can have a profound influence on our own energy patterns. One of the influences that is clearly important relates to our health. If we live or work in an energetically unhealthy environment then we are much more likely to be susceptible to imbalances and disharmonies ourselves.

A practitioner of Chinese medicine who believes that such environmental factors are important in an individual's disharmony pattern, may suggest a referral to a Feng Shui practitioner in order to get advice regarding improving the 'energetic ecology'.

At the moment, such an integration of Chinese practices would be considered very uncommon, but there is no reason to suppose that there will not be a growing interest in considering the environmental health aspects of Chinese medicine built around Feng Shui.

CONCLUSION

As will be apparent from the above discussion, the potential therapeutic avenues that can be explored under the rubric of Chinese medicine are considerable and diverse. Probably the most important point to emerge from this is the realization that the different strands of therapeutic practice are in fact united under a common umbrella of theory and principle.

If you visit an acupuncturist, a Chinese herbalist, an acupressure massage therapist, a Qigong practitioner and so on, you may receive treatments that are very different, but underlying them all is a commonality of purpose, theory and philosophy.

Most practitioners in the West are probably uni-dimensional in that their main area of training is one of the strands – acupuncturist, herbalist and so on. A growing number of practitioners will now hold accredited qualifications in two strands, most commonly herbalism and acupuncture. Some practitioners will have serious interest in other aspects, for example the use of Qigong as a therapeutic tool, in addition to their main specialism.

As the profession of Chinese medicine grows and develops in the West it is not unreasonable to envisage a network of practitioners who would offer the full range of therapeutic interventions. Treatment protocols could thus be more readily customized to the needs of individual patients.

The ideal Chinese medical practice would offer acupuncture, herbal medicine, therapeutic acupressure massage, Qigong classes and treatment, lifestyle and personal counselling and possibly even Feng Shui consultations. All practitioners would be appropriately trained and registered and subject to professional appraisal and development. Such a practice would work in close liaison with conventional Western medical practitioners to offer the best possible forms of treatment for the patients they all work with.

CASE STUDIES

The following brief case studies will not be presented in great detail. The background will be given along with the presenting problems and a Chinese medicine diagnosis will be offered. The focus will then be on discussing the possible approaches to treatment that may be used, either individually or in combination.

Case 1

Presenting Problem

Neil is 18 years old. He went over on his right ankle at a pre-season soccer training session. His ankle is swollen and sore to the touch. He is anxious that he is going to miss the first game of the season in ten days' time. Other than this, Neil is fit and healthy.

Comments

This is a straightforward channel problem. There is no evidence from diagnostic interview of any significant internal disharmony.

Differential Diagnosis

This is a case of Stagnation of Qi and Blood in the Channels due to physical trauma.

Treatment

The principle of treatment is to clear the local stagnation in the channels by moving the Qi and Blood.

It is likely that acupuncture will be used in conjunction with moxabustion over the area of the injury: acupuncture on local channel and 'ashi' points with a reducing manipulation, supplemented by a strong moxa for acute problems. Acupressure massage may also be used to promote Qi and Blood flow through the local area.

Case 2

Presenting Problem

Janet is 68 years old. She is complaining of a dull aching pain that is radiating down the back of her left leg. Occasionally the pain can be acute. This has been a problem that has flared up from time to time over the last ten years. She feels the cold readily and complains of cold back and knees, especially in cold and damp weather.

Comments

This is a combination of an Excess and a Deficient condition. The sciatica problem is likely to be due to Cold–Damp invading the channels of the leg – mainly the Bladder channel. However, other features of the case history suggest an underlying Kidney Yang Deficiency.

Differential Diagnosis

Invasion of the Channels by Cold–Damp and Kidney Yang Deficiency.

Treatment

The principle of treatment would be to expel the Cold–Damp from the channels and to tonify and warm the Kidney Yang.

Acupuncture would be indicated for the channel problem, supplemented by moxabustion on the needle and probably over the low back on a moxa box. Acupuncture can be very effective with the acute Excess symptoms.

The Kidney Yang Deficiency could also be treated by acupuncture and moxabustion, but herbal prescription or patent remedies can also be given. It is likely that a combined treatment with acupuncture and herbs would be effective.

Case 3

Presenting Problem

Anne is 21 years old and is due to be married the next day. She has classic cold symptoms involving shivering with no fever, a general body ache, sneezing and a streaming nose (white/clear discharge).

Comments

Usually the main issue with an invasion by Wind–Cold is to try and ensure the Yin does not transform into the Yang, resulting in Wind–Heat symptom and much more unpleasant symptoms of fever and sore throat and so on.

Differential Diagnosis

Invasion of the Lungs by Wind–Cold.

Treatment

The principle of treatment would be to expel the Wind–Cold from the Lungs and to tonify the Lungs.

Cupping over the Lung area of the back can be very effective in drawing the external pathogenic Wind–Cold from the Lungs. This could be supplemented with acupuncture and/or a herbal prescription.

Case 4

Presenting Problem

George is 45. He has suffered from migraine attacks for many years. When they come on he gets a severe throbbing and pulsating headache above the left eye and over the left temple. The headache is usually accompanied by visual disturbances such as flashing lights and his vision becomes blurred and indistinct, especially in the left eye. When the pain gets really bad he will end up vomiting.

Comments

Case history shows George to be very stressed at work, with a difficult relationship at home. These are classic migraine type symptoms and are invariably associated with a Liver disharmony in Chinese medicine.

Differential Diagnosis

Liver Yang Rising due to Liver Blood/Yin Deficiency. This is a mixed Excess/Deficiency condition.

Treatment

Treatment principle is to subdue the Liver Yang and tonify the Liver Blood/Yin.

The initial treatment will focus on clearing the Yang Excess pattern. Acupuncture with a reducing needling technique is indicated here. George can also be taught some simple self-help acupressure points that he can use (or have someone else use) in the event of an attack feeling imminent.

Herbal prescription can be given to both subdue the Liver Yang and tonify the Liver Blood. Acupuncture and patent herbs may be used together in this instance.

Case 5

Presenting Problem

Agnes was 32 years old. She had suffered from eczema since she was a baby. At the time of consultation she had patches on her arms, her trunk and around her mouth area. The eczema presented as red and itchy and would ooze fluid when scratched. She also had suffered from asthma and an allergic rhinitis usually triggered by pollen and cat hair.

Comments

This is a chronic problem that has created a deficiency in the Lungs and the Kidneys. This was confirmed by other indicators from the diagnostic interview and examination.

Diagnosis

The eczema is a chronic problem of Damp–Heat invading the skin due to the underlying Deficiency of the Lung and Kidney Qi and the invasion of the skin by external Wind.

Treatment

The treatment principle would be to expel the Wind, clear the Damp–Heat and to tonify the Lungs and the Kidneys.

In this instance herbal prescriptions often prove the most effective approach to treatment. Acupuncture may be used, but with skin conditions such as eczema it tends to be less effective than herbal approaches. Treatment is likely to take some considerable time and it may be that acupuncture may be used to supplement the herbal treatment.

Case 6

Presenting Problem

Marie is 27 years old. She has been suffering from a problem of chronic tiredness and lethargy for the last ten months. She is pale and thin and complains of a poor appetite and a bloated abdomen. She finds it very difficult to get up and going in the morning.

Comments

Other indicators in the diagnostic pattern suggest a chronic problem of deficient Qi.

Diagnosis

This presents as a classic example of Spleen Qi Deficiency. In Marie's case it probably relates to poor dietary habits over a long period of time.

Treatment

The treatment principle in this instance will be to tonify the Spleen Qi. Acupuncture and possible herbal treatments may be given. In addition, the patient would be given dietary advice and encouraged to take regular, if limited, mild exercise. The patient may be encouraged to attend a Qigong class once she began to feel a bit better in order to work at promoting the smooth movement of Qi and Blood and to tonify the Kidneys, which underpin the Yin and Yang energy of the body.

8

Chinese Medicine and its Place in Twenty-first-century Health Care

THE CHAPTERS UP to this point have sought to outline the philosophy, theory and systems of Chinese medicine that inform current practitioners in their day-to-day work with patients. However, it is important to look ahead in a somewhat speculative fashion to the role of Chinese medicine in a new and developing paradigm of health-care practice.

I am intending to throw out some ideas, some of which have been articulated in different ways before and some that may not have been. Intuition comes to the fore here and so should it be with anyone reading this chapter. Try not to make an initial judgement. If they don't feel right then reject them, if they sit more comfortably then perhaps you will have a contribution to make in articulating them more fully. Read on with an open mind.

CHINESE MEDICINE TODAY

As we approach the end of the century, there is no doubt that the practices of Chinese medicine are becoming more readily accepted within a Western cultural context. I emphasize the word 'practice' quite deliberately, because while acupuncture, herbal remedies, massage and so on are being embraced as therapies, there is limited evidence that the philosophy and theories are being adopted with open arms. The reasons for this pull in two directions.

On the one hand, acupuncture, herbal medicine and so on, patently work – they bring symptomatic relief and often help with a whole variety of disorders with which Western medical approaches have had limited success. This, of course, has resulted in the rather questionable practice of Western-trained practitioners – doctors, physiotherapists, nurses and so on – learning simplistic symptomatic protocols. For example, simple acupuncture treatment strategies for straightforward problems – usually channel disharmonies – are learned with no understanding of the theory and principles behind them. Now, this is fine as far as it goes, but it has a tendency to lead to a view of acupuncture that is very superficial and that tries to understand its effects in terms of conventionally understood physiological processes. Therefore, as long as Chinese medicine is tolerated at this level then the theory and philosophy will inevitably be kept at arm's length. Only some simple practices will become embraced within Western medicine.

The second problem is implied by the first, but is altogether far more fundamental. If Chinese medicine is adopted in its entirety then this requires that the model of the human being as a subtle energy system also requires to be taken on board. For many Western medical practitioners this, undoubtably, is a bridge too far – at least at this point in time.

The last ten years or so have seen Chinese medicine concentrating on building a professional image and identity within a Western cultural context. This has been absolutely vital. The need to set standards in training, the accreditation of training courses, the adoption of high standards of ethical and professional practice and the move towards registration of practitioners, have all been critical in giving the profession the status and respect that it needs and deserves within Western society. The result is that as the profession as a whole gets its act together and holds itself up to professional scrutiny, then the issue of theory and principles can quite justifiably be placed at the top of the agenda and the implications thoroughly explored.

So, Chinese medicine, certainly in the UK, is at an interesting stage of development, and the nature of the relationship between the Chinese and Western approaches will require that these more fundamental issues be addressed. In China, the two approaches appear as relatively comfortable bedfellows and there seems no reason why this should not happen elsewhere.

TOWARDS AN ENERGY ANATOMY

An excellent and much more technical discussion of the notion of an energy anatomy can be found in the book *Vibrational Medicine* by Richard Gerber MD,[1] but it will be useful to summarize some of the main contributory ideas here. We can look at three energy traditions and see how they may begin to come together:

1. The Human Energy Fields from the Western mystery tradition.
2. The Chakra System of Indian subtle energetics.
3. The Qi and Meridian system of Chinese medicine.

The Human Energy Fields

There is much written about the energy fields that make up the human being. It is suggested that the physical body is merely the densest level of energetic matter that exists within a frequency range that makes it both tangible and visible. There are other 'levels' of energetic matter surrounding the physical with increasingly subtle frequency distributions. Thus, the various levels that are believed to exist are:

- Physical
- Etheric
- Astral
- Mental (containing Instinctive, Intellectual and Spiritual sub-levels)
- Pure Spirit or Causal

Thus, this is diagrammatically shown in Figure 30.

It has also been suggested that the energy distributions at each level are such that there would not be considered to be a distinct or discrete division between them. This is diagrammatically shown in Figure 31.

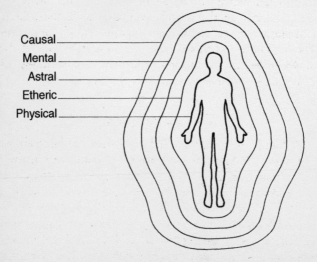

Causal
Mental
Astral
Etheric
Physical

Figure 30. Human energy fields

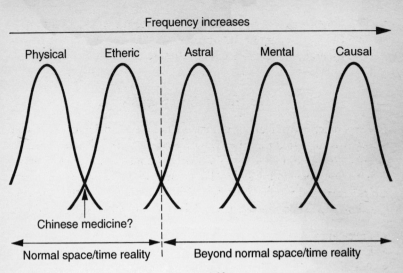

Figure 31. Energy field interactions

Each energy level interacts with its neighbour and it is suggested that the development and organization of the physical body is preceded by stimulation through the higher frequency energy bodies. Thus, in the development of the physical body, the organizational field commences at the Pure Spirit or Causal level, which then creates an organizational matrix at the Mental level, which in turn causes the same to happen at the Astral level, thence at the Etheric level and finally the organizational matrices manifest in physical form – the human body. Thus, and this is where an energetic view of the body dramatically differs from a mechanistic view, energetic organization precedes physical organization, not vice versa!

The Chakra System

The idea of the seven major Chakra centres of the body and the myriad of minor chakras has long been postulated within the Indian spiritual traditions. Ancient Indian texts suggest that the chakras are like energy vortices or centres that exist within our subtle energy levels or bodies and that access directly the cellular structure of the physical body. Chakras may take on the function of 'energy transformers', allowing higher frequency organizational energy fields to function at the relatively lower frequency levels of the physical body. Each major chakra appears associated with a particular gland of

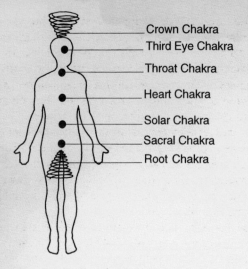

Figure 32. The Chakra system

the endocrine system giving access to the hormonal flows and changes in the body. The Chakra body is shown in Figure 32.

It is suggested that the chakras are connected to each other and link through the body by subtle energetic channels called 'nadis'. It is tempting to suggest that the chakras and the nadis are simply an alternative nomenclature for the acupuncture points and the meridian system, but the literature suggests that they function at a more subtle level than the meridian system and may, in effect, complement it.

The work of the medical intuitive, Caroline Myss,[2] demonstrates that thought processes and emotional reactions are clearly associated with each of the chakras and that imbalances or blockages in the energy flow associated with the chakras can directly result in physical illness. She describes illness as being a function of how much time we have tied up in our cell tissue, thus pointing clearly to the fact that more subtle energy processes, which exist outside a conventional space–time framework, can directly impinge on the physical body through the interaction with the chakra system.

The Qi Energy and Meridian System

The third 'anatomical' part of our energy system is that articulated in the theory of Chinese medicine. It seems that the Qi flow and the meridian or channel networks operate at the cusp between the physical and the non-tangible energetic system. Thus, as the etheric body is seen to be closest to the physical, the meridians may be seen as forming what Richard Gerber calls the 'physical–etheric interface'. Thus, the Qi energy of the universe enters through the etheric energy level, accessing the body through the major and minor acupuncture points and flowing to the cellular structures via the energy gradients and concentrations that we term the meridian system.

Thus, when a disharmony appears in the body, for whatever reason, it has firstly manifested itself at the etheric level and probably at more subtle energetic levels before that. Physical illness comes at the end of a chain of energetic processes that probably involve imbalances that enter through the chakra and nadis system as well as imbalances that enter through the meridian system.

It is a well-known fact that there are changes in skin resistance at acupuncture points on the body and that this can be used to facilitate point location in Chinese medicine. It has thus been erroneously assumed that the meridians represent an electromagnetic network and that this will eventually provide the conventional explanation of what happens in acupuncture.

More recent research funded through the Dove Healing Trust by Julian Kenyon[3] seems to be pointing to a quite unique dimension of energetic scalar fields quite separate from conventional electromagnetic fields.

SO, HOW MIGHT CHINESE MEDICINE WORK?

As was pointed out early on in the book, Chinese medicine has evolved as an essentially empirical science, where effects were recorded and explanations offered in terms of the basic principles. Now, as a therapeutic endeavour this serves very well and will continue to do so, but as we move towards really addressing what energy medicine is all about, questions will be raised as to what is actually going on at an energetic level when an acupuncture needle is inserted into the body, or when a particular herbal remedy is given and so on.

If we can accept the notion that the body is essentially an energetic network that oscillates at different frequencies, then perhaps some hypotheses can be entertained.

The various energetic oscillations will correspond to the physical and the non-physical aspects of our being. Some of it, like our skin, bones, muscles, blood supply and organs we can see, touch and directly interact with. Other aspects, such as our chakras, our meridian system and our Qi flow we cannot see, touch or directly interact with, but we infer their reality through the subtle effects of practices such as Chinese medicine.

As has been suggested before, when our bodies experience an illness or disharmony, this will initially develop in the organizational energy matrices. This energy matrix will be made up of a highly complex multitude of frequency interactions. Rupert Sheldrake,[4] a plant biologist, has promoted the highly controversial view of all living systems being defined in their growth and developmental patterns by organizational matrices which he calls 'morphogenetic fields'. When an illness develops this may be considered as a 'blip' in the matrix and if the illness becomes chronic, then the 'blip' becomes more established in the field and it becomes progressively less likely that the original 'healthy' matrix will re-establish itself.

So, if a patient comes to a practitioner of Chinese medicine with a particular disharmony, the practitioner may suggest acupuncture. When the needles are inserted into the appropriate acupuncture points they may set up some form of sympathetic harmonic frequency response in the energetic field or matrix. The result of this process will be to begin to reorganize the energetic matrix back towards its initial 'healthy' structure. As the energetic structure is restored to normal, there will be a consequent 'knock on' effect at the physical level resulting in the relief of symptoms and the re-balancing of the original disharmony.

An analogy may help here. When a tuning fork is struck it sets up a series of sympathetic harmonic oscillations that can have a dramatic physical consequence if the phase and frequency are correct, for example it may shatter a glass.

Thus, Chinese medicine may well be working by influencing the organizational energy matrix through the medium of stimulating frequencies in the Qi flow of the body, which in turn interact with the energy levels initially through the physical–etheric interface described by Richard Gerber.

CAN IT ALL HANG TOGETHER?

It is my belief that we are at the beginning of a process that will articulate in quite specific terms the nature of the human energetic anatomy system. I am suggesting that the three systems outlined very briefly above will form a central part of a process that begins to draw together a deep understanding of how, as human beings, we are much more than a physical body, but in reality highly complex multidimensional energy beings, who in some aspects cross not only frequency dimensions but also space–time dimensions as well.

Some of the more exciting and controversial claims of Qigong healing, for example, suggest that the effects can be experienced independent of space and time. In other words, the Qigong healer neither needs to be physically or temporally adjacent to the patient being worked with. This seems very similar to that which is reported in cases of absent and distance healing.

This whole area remains one of hypothesis, speculation, debate and controversy. However, if the ideas of an energy medicine are to be taken seriously then this is a debate that scientists, practitioners and patients require to engage in actively. Chinese medicine, with its long history and proven track record as a therapeutic tool, must be a central plank of this emerging new paradigm. It undoubtably has the most clearly articulated energetic anatomy and physiology system currently developed. It appears to operate at the very interface between the physical energetic level and the non-physical energetic levels. As such, it is of crucial importance in understanding these processes and in building a new therapeutic paradigm for the twenty-first century.

The ideas and hypotheses developed in this final chapter are largely personal and the whole story will be much, much more complex and amazing than I have been able to suggest here. If at the end of the day, this book has been able to inform and excite you about Chinese medicine and suggest its place in the developing health-care paradigm for the future, then it will have more than done its job.

Notes

An Introduction to Chinese Medicine

1. Confucius quoted in D. Bensky and A. Gamble, *Chinese Herbal Medicine – A Materia Medica*, Eastland Press, Seattle, 1993, p. 3.
2. *Yellow Emperor's Inner Classic*, People's Press, Beijing, 1963.
3. 'The Systematic Classic of Acupuncture & Moxabustion' quoted in J. O'Connor and D. Bensky, *Acupuncture: A Comprehensive Text*, Eastland Press, Seattle, 1981.
4. 'The Divine Husbandman's Classic of the Materia Medica' quoted in D. Bensky and A. Gamble, *Chinese Herbal Medicine – A Materia Medica*, Eastland Press, Seattle, 1993.

Chapter 2: The Basic Substances

1. Ted Kaptchuk, *Chinese Medicine: The Web that Has No Weaver*, Rider, London, 1983, p. 35.

Chapter 8: Chinese Medicine and its Place in Twenty-first-century Health Care

1. Richard Gerber, *Vibrational Medicine*, Bear & Co, Santa Fe, 1988.
2. Carolyn Myss (and Norman Shealy), *The Creation of Health*, Stillpoint, Walpole, NH, 1988.
3. Julian Kenyon, *Caduceus*, Issue 19, 1993, p. 10.
4. Rupert Sheldrake, *The Presence of the Past*, Collins, London, 1988.

Appendix: Solutions to Exercises

YIN AND YANG EXERCISE

The following are my suggested solutions to the simple exercise on Yin and Yang that was given at the end of the Chapter 1.

	Situation	Yin or Yang?	Change
1.	A rowdy school classroom	Yang	Teacher sets the class work.
2.	A parked car	Yin	Get in and drive off.
3.	A block of ice	Yin	Heat it and melt it.
4.	A thumping migraine headache	Yang	Take an analgesic.
5.	An incomplete jigsaw puzzle	Yin	Complete puzzle.
6.	A golfer lining up a putt	Yin	Putt the ball.
7.	A bout of diarrhoea	Yang	Take appropriate medication.
8.	An aeroplane taking off	Yang	Aeroplane in cruise flight.
9.	A politician delivering a speech	Yang	Politician stops talking (cheers!)
10.	A hard-boiled egg	Yin	Roll it down the hill.
11.	A raw egg	Yin	Boil it.
12.	A CD of a heavy metal rock band	Yin	Play it!
13.	A Mozart piano sonata being played	Yang	Stop playing the piano.
14.	A runner at the end of a marathon	Yang	Runner at start of marathon.
15.	A coin	Yin	Spend it.
16.	A game of chess	Yin	Start playing.
17.	A packet of sherbet dip	Yin	Suck the sherbet.
18.	A car that has run out of petrol	Yin	Fill it up and start the engine.
19.	A book	Yin	Read it.
20.	Someone performing a Taiqi exercise	Yang	Perform static Qigong posture.
21.	A baby with colic	Yang	Settle baby with a feed.
22.	A hot summer's day	Yang	Summer night.
23.	A yawn	Yang	Go to sleep!
24.	A video of an aerobic exercise	Yin	Follow the video exercise.
25.	Your thought processes at this minute	Who knows!	Only you know!

WHAT PATTERNS CAN YOU SEE?

Suggested solution to the case study given at the end of Chapter 6.

General Considerations

In this case study there are various factors about the general situation that are worth pointing out.

1. Maria is a physiotherapist and is likely to be engaged in some quite heavy physical work from time to time.
2. She has a demanding position at work and is under a lot of pressure as a result of her promotion.
3. She is in an extremely stressful situation as a result of the breakdown of her marriage, which appears very difficult and acrimonious.
4. Her dietary patterns are not good.
5. Her emotional pattern is very moody and irritable.

So, What Is Going On?

It is likely that the major predisposing problem is one of stress, both from her work and from her family situation. This has caused her Liver Qi to become stagnant. This is suggested by the pattern of her emotional outbursts, worse prior to a period, the feeling of throat constriction and the wiry pulse.

In addition it is likely that the Liver has invaded the Spleen, which in itself is likely to be deficient due to irregular and inconsistent dietary habits. This will produce Qi deficient symptoms such as feeling bloated, heavy legs and general lethargy. The slight toothmarking also suggests Spleen Qi deficient.

So the diagnosis would be:

Liver Qi Stagnation (Excess Pattern) and Spleen Qi Deficiency (Deficient Pattern)

The treatment principle would be to promote the smooth flow of Liver Qi and to tonify the Spleen. Maria would have to adopt a more balanced dietary pattern and it may be recommended that she take counselling to help her through her marital break up. As far as Chinese medicine is concerned, acupuncture and/or herbal remedies would be appropriate in this instance.

Bibliography

The following bibliography is by no means comprehehensive, but it does offer a good source guide for further study.

CHINESE MEDICINE – GENERAL

Beinfield, H. and Korngold, E., *'Between Heaven & Earth'*, Ballantine, New York, 1991.

Kaptchuk, Ted, *Chinese Medicine: The Web that Has No Weaver*, Rider, London, 1983.

Maciocia, Giovanni, *The Foundations of Chinese Medicine*, Churchill Livingstone, London, 1989.

Maciocia, Giovanni, *The Practice of Chinese Medicine*, Churchill Livingstone, London, 1994.

Wiseman, Ellis and Zmiewski, *The Fundamentals of Chinese Medicine*, Paradigm, Brookline, 1985.

ACUPUNCTURE

Connelly, Dianne, *Traditional Acupuncture: The Law of Five Elements*, Centre for Traditional Acupuncture, Columbia, 1979.

Mole, Peter, *Acupuncture*, Element Books, Shaftesbury, 1991.

O'Connor, J. and Bensky, D., *Acupuncture: A Comprehensive Text*, Eastland, Seattle, 1981.

CHINESE HERBAL MEDICINE

Bensky, D. and Barolet R., *Chinese Herbal Medicine, Formulas & Strategies*, Eastland, Seattle, 1993.

Bensky, D. and Gamble, A., *Chinese Herbal Medicine, Materia Medica*, Eastland Press, Seattle, 1993.

Fratkin, J., *Chinese Herbal Patent Formulas*, Shya, Boulder, 1986.

CHINESE DIETARY THERAPY

Flaws, B. and Wolfe, H., *Prince Wen Hui's Cookbook*, Paradigm, Massachusetts, 1983.

TAIQI AND QIGONG

Klein, B., *Movements of Magic*, Newcastle, California, 1984.
Lam Kam Chuen, *The Way of Energy*, Gaia, London, 1991.
Liang, T.T., *T'ai Chi Chuan for Health & Self Defence*, Vintage, New York, 1977.
McRitchie, J., *Chi Kung*, Element Books, Shaftesbury, 1993.
Reid, H., *The Way of Harmony*, Gaia, London, 1988.
Wong Kiew Kit, *The Art of Chi Kung*, Element Books, Shaftesbury, 1993.

CHINESE PHILOSOPHY

Hua-Ching Ni, *I Ching, The Book of Changes*, Eternal Breath of Tao, Santa Monica, 1992.
Mitchell, Stephen (trans), *Tao Te Ching*, Harper Perennial, New York, 1991.

GENERAL HEALTH CARE

Gerber, Richard, *Vibrational Medicine*, Bear & Co, Santa Fe, 1988.
Myss, C. and Shealy, N., 'The Creation of Health*, Stillpoint, Walpole, NH, 1988.

Glossary

Acupressure: Works on the same basic principle as acupuncture, but the Qi is worked on by pressure and massage instead of needles.

Acupuncture: The treatment in Chinese medicine where the Qi flow in the body is influenced by the insertion of fine needles into specific points in the body.

An Mo: The Chinese for massage. Literally 'push' and 'rub'.

Blood: The Chinese concept of Blood differs from the western view.

Chakra: One of the energy centres of the body. Based on the Indian understanding of the energy body.

Channel: The series of pathways in which the Qi flow through the body is concentrated (see also **Meridians**).

Chong Mai: The penetrating vessel; one of the eight extraordinary meridians.

Cupping: A treatment technique involving drawing the Qi and Blood to the surface of the skin using a vacuum created inside a glass or bamboo cup.

Dai Mai: The girdle vessel; one of the eight extraordinary Meridians.

Dan Tien: Energy centres in the body. There are considered to be three, an upper (between eyebrows); a middle (in the centre of the trunk); the lower (in the lower abdomen). Qi is considered as being stored there.

Dao/Daoism: Chinese philosophical and spiritual system. Dao literally means 'the way'. Sometimes spelt as 'Tao'. See *Tao Te Ching* by Lao Tzu.

Dayan Qigong: Wild goose Qigong form. A sequence of moving exercises based on the movements of wild geese.

Du Mai: The governing vessel; one of the eight extraordinary Meridians.

Eight Principle Patterns: The system of organizing diagnostic information in Chinese medicine according to the principles of Yin, Yang; Interior, Exterior; Hot, Cold; Excess, Deficiency.

Empty Heat: Internal heat in the body resulting from a deficiency of Yin.

Energy Bodies: The energy 'sheaths' that are considered to surround the physical body.

External: In Chinese medicine any factors influencing the body from outside.

Extra Fu: Less important 'minor' organs in Chinese medicine.

143

Feng Shui: The Chinese system of analysing the energy patterns of the physical environment.

Five Elements/Phases: The system in Chinese medicine based on observations of the natural world. System built around the elements of water, wood, fire, metal and earth.

Five Palm Sweat: Characteristic sweat associated with Yin deficiency appearing on the palms, the soles of the feet and the chest.

Four Levels: System for diagnosis in Chinese medicine.

Fu: The hollow Yang organs of the body.

Gan: Sweet. Used to assign taste to Chinese herbs.

Gu Qi: The Qi extracted in the Stomach through the digestion of food and drink.

Hegu: The acupuncture point Large Intestine 4. Translates as 'Tiger's Mouth'.

Internal: Refers to aspects of disharmonies that arise within the body.

Jiao: Refers to the areas of the body. 'Heater' or 'Burner'.

Jin Ye: Body fluids. Jin refers to the lighter fluids; Ye refers to the denser fluids.

Jing: The essence of all life in the body. The energy that governs our development.

Jing Luo Zhi Qi: Qi flowing through the Meridians.

Jue Yin: Arm and leg Channels of the Pericardium and the Liver.

Ke Cycle: The cycle of mutual control in the Five Element system.

Kong Qi: Qi derived in the Lungs from the air.

Ku: Bitter. Term used to describe taste of Chinese herbs.

Laogong: Acupuncture point in the centre of the palm – Pericardium 8. Literally translates as 'Labour Palace'.

Luo: The system of connecting channels between the major channels.

Marrow: The substance that makes up the brain and the spinal column in Chinese medicine.

Materia Medica: The complete description of all Chinese herbs.

Meridian: See **Channels**.

Mingmen Fire: The nature of the essential warming energy of Kidney Yang. Considered to be vital in maintaining the heat in the body.

Moxabustion: The treatment approach involving the burning of Chinese herb, moxa. Moxa is made from a species of mugwort – *Artemisia vulgaris*.

Phlegm: A disharmony of the body fluids produces either external or visible phlegm, or internal or invisible phlegm.

Post-Natal/After Heaven Qi/Jing: Qi or Jing manufactured from air or food.

Pre-Natal/Before Heaven Qi/Jing: Qi or Jing passed on from our parents.

Qi (Chi): The essential energy of the universe which is fundamental to all aspects of life. Permeates the whole body. Concentrates in the channels.

Qigong (Chi Kung): Literally translates as 'energy cultivation'. A series of moving and static exercises designed for this function.

Qihai: The 'Sea of Qi' in the lower Dantian. The acupuncture point Ren 6.

Qi Ni: Rebellious Qi. Qi that moves in the 'wrong' direction.

Qi Xian: Sinking Qi. Qi sinks when it is too deficient to perform its holding function.

Qi Xu: Deficient Qi.

Qi Zhi: Stagnant Qi. Qi that has become sluggish and which ceases to move properly.

Quchi: Acupuncture point Large Intestine 11. Literally translates as 'crooked pool'.

Ren Mai: The conception vessel, one of the eight extraordinary Meridians.

San Jiao: The Triple Warmer/Heater/Burner. A process organ in the Chinese Zangfu system.

Sea of Marrow: The Chinese believe the brain is composed of Marrow, which is then called the 'sea'.

Semen Palace: The male source of sexual energy in the Lower Dantian.

Shao Yang: San Jiao and Gall Bladder channels.

Shao Yin: Heart and Kidney channels.

Shen: An important aspect of mind or spirit in Chinese medicine.

Sheng Cycle: The cycle of mutual production or promotion in the Five Element system Chinese medicine.

Six Stage Patterns: A diagnostic system in Chinese medicine.

Suan: Sour. A description of taste for Chinese herbs.

Taiqi: Literally translates as 'the supreme ultimate'. Usually refers to the martial form of moving practice which should properly be termed Taiqiquan - Supreme Ultimate Fist or Boxing Art (sometimes written as T'ai Chi Chaun).

Tai Yang: The Small Intestine and Bladder channels.

Tai Yin: The Lung and Spleen channels.

Three Treasures: The collective term used to describe Qi, Jing and Shen.

Wei Qi: Defensive Qi which protects the body from invasion by External Pathogenic Factors. It flows just beneath the skin.

Xian: Salty. A description of taste for Chinese herbs.

Xin: Acrid. A description of taste for Chinese herbs.

Xu: Deficiency. A common disharmony in Chinese medicine.

Xue: The Chinese for Blood.

Yang: One aspect of the complementary opposites in Chinese philosophy. Reflects the more active, moving, warmer aspects.

Yang Ming: Large Intestine and Stomach channels.

Yin: One aspect of the complementary opposites in Chinese philosophy. Reflects the more passive, still, reflective, aspects.

Ying Qi: Nutritive aspects of Qi that nourish the body.

Yuan Qi: Original or source Qi. That aspect of Qi passed on from our parents.

Zang: The solid Yin organs of the body.

Zangfu: The complete Yin and Yang organs of the body.

Zangfu Zhi Qi: Qi of the organs. The Qi that nourishes the organs of the body.

Zheng Qi: Normal or upright Qi. Qi that circulates through the channels and the organs of the body.

Zong Qi: Gathering Qi. The Qi that gathers in the chest area through the coming together of Gu Qi and Kong Qi.

Useful Addresses

It is important when considering Chinese medicine as a form of treatment that any prospective patient can be sure that they can access a reputable, registered practitioner. This is best done through a professional association or council.

The author would be delighted to hear from any interested reader who would like to obtain further information regarding Chinese medicine. He can be contacted at the following address: The Kun Chen Clinic, 34 Orchard Drive, Giffnock, Glasgow G46 7NU, Scotland, tel. and fax. 0141 638 8801.

AUSTRALIA

Acupuncture Ethics and Standards Organization, PO Box 84, Merrylands, New South Wales 2160.

Australian Natural Therapists Association, PO Box 308, Melrose Park, South Australia 5039. Tel. 8297 9533. Fax. 8297 0003.

Qigong Association of Australia, 458 White Horse Road, Surrey Hills, Victoria 3127. Tel. 03 836 6961.

The National Herbalists Association of Australia, 247–9 Kingsgrove Road, Kingsgrove, South Australia 2208.

NEW ZEALAND

New Zealand Natural Health Practitioners Accreditation Board, PO Box 37–491, Auckland. Tel. 9625 9966.

New Zealand Register of Acupuncturists, PO Box 9950, Wellington 1.

The New Zealand College of Naturopathic Medicine, Christchurch.

Useful Addresses

UK

The Council for Acupuncture, 179 Gloucester Place, London NW1 6DX. Tel. 0171 724 5756. Fax. 0171 724 5330.

The Kun Chen Clinic, 34 Orchard Drive, Giffnock, Glasgow G46 7NU. Tel. and fax. 0141 638 8801.

The Register of Chinese Herbal Medicine, 21 Warbeck Road, London W12 8NS.

The Register of Traditional Chinese Medicine, 19 Trinity Road, London N2 8JJ. Tel. 0181 883 8431.

USA

American Association of Acupuncture and Oriental Medicine, National Acupuncture Headquarters, 1424 16th Street NW, Suite 501, Washington DC 20036.

American Herb Association, Box 353, Rescue, California 96672.

China Advocates, 1635 Irving Street, San Francisco, California 94122. Tel. 415 665 4505.

Qi Gong Resource Associates, 1755 Homet Road, Pasadena, California 91106. Tel. 818 564 9751.

Qigong Academy, 8103 Marlborough Avenue, Cleveland, Ohio 44129. Tel. 216 842 9628.

Qigong Human Life Research Foundation, PO Box 5327, Cleveland, Ohio 44101. Tel. 216 475 4712.

The Qigong Institute, East West Academy of Healing Arts, 450 Sutter Street, Suite 916, San Francisco, California 94108. Tel. 415 788 2227/323 1221.

The American Herbalists Guild, PO Box 1127, Forestville, California 95436.

Traditional Acupuncture Clinic, America City Building, Suite 100, Columbia, Maryland 210044. Tel. 301 596 6006.

Index

Index

emotions 47–8, 54, 55, 60–2, 68–9, 78–9
energy fields 132–3
energy patterns 77
environment 69, 124
Excess 107–8
exercise 67, 123
Extra Fu 45, 58
eyes 54–5, 75

face 72
fear 51, 62
Feng Shui 124
Fire 12–13, 64–5
Five Elements/Phases 9–14
Fu (Yang organs) 45, 56–8, 103–4

Gall Bladder 56
grief 61
growth 21, 49
Gu Qi 18, 23–4, 56
gynaecological patterns 79

hair 51, 52–3, 72
head 75
hearing and smelling 74
Heart 46–8, 55, 94–6
Heart 64–5
    Deficient 89
    Excess 89
    Exterior 88
    in Blood 26
herbal remedies 115–16

Jin 28
Jing 21–3, 30, 31, 37, 49
    Post-Natal/After Heaven 21
    Pre-Natal/Congenital/Before Heaven 21, 66
Jing Ye 26
joy 47, 55, 61

Ke Cycle 12–13
Kidneys 14, 21–2, 49–51, 62, 101–3

Large Intestine 57
lifestyle 66, 79, 122–4
limbs 48
Liver 53–5, 61, 98–101
looking 72–3
Lower Jiao 50
Lungs 51–3, 61, 91–4

Marrow 22, 23, 24, 50, 58
Materia Medica 3, 115
meridian system 32–42, 134–5
Mingmen Fire 50
Mother and Son cycle 10
mouth 48
moxabustion 112–13
muscles 48

nails 54
nose 53, 75

pain 77–8, 80
palpation 80
pensiveness 61
Pericardium 42, 45, 55
Phlegm 64
process 6, 17, 33, 43–4, 55
pulse 81–4

Qi 17–20, 26, 28–9, 30, 31, 32–4, 38–42, 49, 51–2, 54, 134–5
    Post-Natal/After Heaven 18
    Pre-Natal/Before Heaven 18, 66
Qigong 2, 41–2, 67, 116–20
questioning 74–9

relationships 122
Ren Mai 40, 41
reproduction 21, 49
respiration 51–2

sadness 61
San Jiao 28, 37, 45, 57
sexual activity 67
Shamanism 2
Shen 25, 29–30, 31, 46–7
Sheng Cycle 10–12